Note to the Reader

Dear Reader,

Welcome to the immersive world of "Steam & Sauna: A Concise Guidebook". This book is not just a traditional read; it's an invitation to explore the history, science, and health benefits of saunas and steam in a way that suits your unique journey. Picture it as a catalog of ideas, a companion meant to be enjoyed at random while basking in the soothing warmth of a steam or sauna session.

Feel free to dive into the chapters that pique your interest, whether it's the historical evolution of saunas, the science behind their therapeutic effects, or the profound impact on health and wellness. This book is designed to be as flexible as your sauna or steam experience – read it leisurely, skip around, or use it as a reference guide as you embark on your exploration of integrating steam and sauna into your life and home.

May these pages serve as a source of inspiration and knowledge, providing you with a foundation to understand and appreciate the rich tapestry of traditions and innovations woven into the world of saunas and steam. Whether you're a seasoned enthusiast or just beginning your journey, let this book be your companion, guiding you through the myriad benefits and possibilities that these age-old practices bring to modern living.

Wishing you warmth, relaxation, and boundless discovery,

Alberto Rossi,
11/2023

Acknowledgment

In the exploration of saunas and steam within these pages, I am grateful for the invaluable insights and leadership provided by SaunaFin (Toronto, Ontario, Canada). Their rich expertise in the contemporary world of high-end sauna and steam installation has been a guiding light in the creation of this book. As pioneers in the industry, SaunaFin's commitment to quality and innovation aligns seamlessly with the spirit of our narrative. Their contributions have not only enriched the content but also served as a testament to the enduring legacy of sauna traditions. I extend my sincere appreciation for their collaborative spirit and dedication to elevating the understanding of these ancient practices in our modern world. For more on SaunaFin, please see the Afterword at the end of this Book.

SAUNA & STEAM
A CONCISE GUIDEBOOK

ISBN
978-1-989647-33-2

A Byrd Press Publication
Toronto
www.byrdpress.com
publisher@byrdpress.com

Art Direction Paulo Santinelli

SAUNA & STEAM
A CONCISE GUIDEBOOK

Dedicated to Galen of Pergamon

Galen of Pergamon, a towering figure in ancient medicine during the 2nd century AD, made enduring contributions to the field through his prolific writings and empirical approach. Serving as a physician to Roman emperors, including Marcus Aurelius, Galen's achievements encompassed anatomy, physiology, and pathology. Notably, he advocated for the therapeutic benefits of baths, aligning with the Roman tradition of communal bathing. Galen emphasized the healing properties of hot baths, considering them instrumental in maintaining health and preventing illness. His advocacy for bathing practices reflected the broader cultural significance of communal baths in ancient Rome, combining hygiene with social interactions. Galen's influence extended far beyond his time, shaping medical thought for centuries and highlighting the enduring importance of his contributions to both theory and practice in the ancient world.

Table of Contents

Sauna

Steam

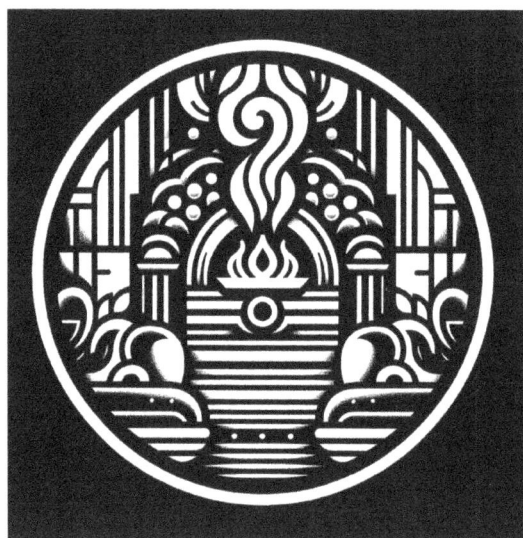

1. Sauna: The Essentials

A sauna is a designated space or room specifically crafted to facilitate dry or wet heat sessions, typically maintained at temperatures ranging from 70 to 100 degrees Celsius (158 to 212 degrees Fahrenheit). Renowned for its cultural significance, saunas are associated with relaxation, social interaction, and diverse health advantages.

Historical Roots:
The origins of the sauna trace back to Finland, where this practice has been an integral part of the culture for centuries. The term "sauna" itself is of Finnish origin. Early iterations of saunas likely involved simple pits dug into hillsides, evolving over time into the wooden structures that have become synonymous with saunas.

The traditional Finnish sauna experience involves heating a confined space using a wood-burning stove or rocks. Water is then poured over the heated rocks, generating steam and creating a hot and humid environment within the sauna. This is typically followed by a refreshing plunge into a cold lake or snow, constituting a customary cooling-off process.

Global Influence and Modern Varieties:
The concept of the sauna has transcended its Finnish origins, permeating various cultures globally. Today, saunas exist in diverse forms and styles. The different types include:

1. **Traditional Finnish Sauna:** Utilizes a wood-burning stove or electric heater, with water poured over rocks to produce steam for a holistic experience.

2. **Infrared Sauna:** Incorporates infrared heaters emitting light absorbed by the skin, offering an alternative heat experience compared to traditional saunas.

3. **Steam Room:** Creates a humid environment with high humidity levels through a steam generator, providing a distinct sensory experience.

4. **Dry Sauna:** Typically electrically heated, emitting dry heat without the introduction of steam, contributing to a more arid atmosphere.

Health and Wellness Benefits:
Saunas are often associated with a range of health benefits, though individual experiences may vary.

Some potential advantages include:

- **Relaxation:** Saunas are recognized for their ability to induce relaxation and alleviate stress.

- **Enhanced Circulation:** The heat generated in saunas promotes increased blood flow, contributing to improved circulation.

- **Detoxification:** Sweating induced by the sauna is thought by some to aid in the elimination of toxins from the body.

- **Muscle and Joint Well-being:** The soothing heat in saunas can offer relief from muscle and joint discomfort.

Before incorporating sauna sessions into a routine, it is advisable to seek guidance from healthcare professionals, particularly for individuals with pre-existing health conditions.

Sauna: Cultural Significance

Saunas hold significant cultural importance across various societies, each imbuing this practice with unique rituals, social dynamics, and meanings. Here's a detailed overview of the significance of saunas in different cultures:

1. Finnish Culture:

Historical Roots: The sauna is deeply ingrained in Finnish culture, with roots tracing back thousands of years. It is considered a place for physical and spiritual cleansing.

Social Gathering: Saunas are central to Finnish social life, offering a space for family bonding, community discussions, and even business meetings.

Rites of Passage: Saunas play a role in various rites of passage, such as celebrating milestones like weddings, births, and even funerals.

2. Japanese *Onsen* Culture:

Natural Hot Springs: In Japan, hot springs or *"onsen"* play a role similar to saunas. The emphasis is on communal bathing, relaxation, and a connection with nature.

Cleansing Rituals: Japanese culture views bathing as a form of purification. The *onsen* experience is often seen as a way to cleanse the body and soul.

3. Russian Banya Tradition:

Bathing as a Ritual: In Russia, the *banya* is a traditional sauna, and the experience involves a series of rituals, including beating oneself or others with birch branches for a rejuvenating effect.

Social Aspect: Similar to Finnish saunas, the Russian *banya* is a social space where friends and family come together, fostering connections.

4. Turkish Hammam Culture:

Cleansing and Socializing: The Turkish *hammam* is a place for both physical and spiritual cleansing. It also serves as a social hub where people come together for discussions and relaxation.

Architectural Beauty: *Hammams* are often intricately designed, reflecting the cultural emphasis on beauty and aesthetics.

5. Native American Sweat Lodge:

Spiritual Cleansing: Various Native American tribes practice sweat lodge ceremonies for spiritual and physical purification. Rocks are heated, and water infused with herbs is poured over them to create steam.

Community Connection: The sweat lodge is a communal experience, reinforcing a sense of community and shared spirituality.

6. Korean *Jjimjilbang* Tradition:

Sauna and Beyond: *Jjimjilbangs* are Korean bathhouses that often include saunas. These establishments serve as more than just places for bathing, offering diverse amenities like sleeping rooms and entertainment spaces.

24/7 Culture: *Jjimjilbangs* are known for being open 24/7, allowing people to visit at any time for relaxation, socializing, and even overnight stays.

7. Scandinavian Sauna Culture:

Hygge **and Well-being:** In Scandinavian countries, saunas are integral to the concept of "*hygge*," representing a cozy and content way of life. Saunas contribute to overall well-being and a sense of comfort.

Across these diverse cultures, the sauna experience extends beyond mere heat therapy; it encompasses social bonding, spiritual rituals, and a holistic approach to health and well-being. The significance of saunas is deeply woven into the fabric of each culture, reflecting the values and traditions of the people who practice them.

The primary difference between steam rooms and saunas lies in the type of heat they provide and the resulting atmospheric conditions.

Steam Room:

Heat Source: Steam rooms generate heat by boiling water and releasing steam into the enclosed space.

Humidity: Steam rooms are characterized by high humidity levels, as the primary element is moisture-laden steam.

Temperature: The temperature in a steam room typically ranges between 40 to 50 degrees Celsius (104 to 122 degrees Fahrenheit).

Experience: The moist heat in a steam room can create a sensation of warmth that penetrates the skin, and many find it invigorating for respiratory health.

Sauna:

Heat Source: Saunas, on the other hand, use dry heat generated by heating rocks or an electric stove. Water can be poured over the heated rocks to create steam, but the overall atmosphere remains much drier than in a steam room.

Humidity: Saunas have lower humidity levels compared to steam rooms, with the emphasis on dry heat.

Temperature: Sauna temperatures are higher, typically ranging from 70 to 100 degrees Celsius (158 to 212 degrees Fahrenheit).

Experience: Saunas offer a dry heat experience, and the higher temperatures can induce profuse sweating, promoting detoxification and muscle relaxation.

As for the notion of writing this book with separate "steam" and "sauna" discreet sections, or books-within-the-book, it's possible that these topics could be exploring various aspects related to wellness practices, but utilizing different means and coming from different engineering, cultural and wellness practice.

1. Diversity of Experiences: The decision to write about steam rooms in one book and saunas in another could be driven by a desire to explore the unique characteristics and benefits of each experience. This allows for a comprehensive exploration of the diverse ways in which individuals pursue relaxation and well-being.

2. Cultural Significance: Since steam rooms and saunas hold cultural significance in various societies, separate books could delve into the cultural practices, rituals, and historical backgrounds associated with each, providing readers with a more in-depth understanding of the cultural context.

3. Wellness and Health Focus: The books might focus on the distinct wellness and health benefits associated with steam rooms and saunas, respectively. Each environment has its unique therapeutic properties, and dedicating separate books allows for a thorough examination of these benefits.

4. Practical Guidance: The books may also provide practical guidance on how to incorporate steam rooms or saunas into one's lifestyle, addressing considerations such as frequency, duration, and potential health precautions.

In essence, the decision to write separate books on steam rooms and saunas stems from our desire to offer a nuanced exploration of each experience, considering their unique characteristics, cultural contexts, and potential health and wellness benefits.

With this in mind, let's start with Sauna.

2. Ancient Beginnings
Early Sauna-Like Practices

Ancient beginnings of sauna-like practices can be traced back to various cultures, showcasing a rich history of heat bathing rituals that served both practical and ceremonial purposes. Here are glimpses into the early sauna-like practices across different regions:

1. Ancient China:

In ancient China, stove-based bathing was a unique and innovative practice that emerged around 2000 BCE. This early form of heat bathing represented an early precursor to what would later develop into various sauna-like practices. Here's a closer exploration of stove-based bathing in ancient China:

1. Origin and Early References:
• Stove-based bathing in ancient China has its roots in the Xia and Shang dynasties (around 2000-1046 BCE).
• Early historical texts, such as the "Er Ya" dictionary (3rd century BCE), make references to the use of heated stones for bathing.

2. Stove-Based Bathing Process:
• The process typically involved creating a chamber or room where stones were heated.
• Large stones were placed in a specific area, often in the center of the bathing space.
• These stones were heated through the combustion of wood or other fuels.

3. Design of Bathing Chambers:
• The bathing chambers were constructed with materials conducive to retaining heat, such as clay or stone.
• Walls were built to enclose the space and contain the heat generated by the heated stones.

4. Usage and Purpose:
• Stove-based bathing in ancient China served both practical and therapeutic purposes.
• Individuals would enter the heated chamber to experience the warmth and potential health benefits.

5. Therapeutic Significance:
• Similar to later sauna practices, stove-based bathing was believed to have therapeutic effects on the body.

- The heat was thought to promote relaxation, relieve muscular tension, and potentially offer detoxification through sweating.

6. Cultural Context:
- The practice of stove-based bathing was likely influenced by Chinese notions of balance and harmony in the body.
- The concept of balancing "yin" and "yang" energies, fundamental to Chinese philosophy, may have played a role in the perceived health benefits of stove-based bathing.

7. Evolution of Bathing Practices:
- Over time, the stove-based bathing practices in China evolved, contributing to the broader tradition of Chinese bathing culture.
- The development of bathhouses and public bathing facilities became more sophisticated in subsequent dynasties.

8. Influence on Chinese Medicine:
- The principles of traditional Chinese medicine, which emphasizes the balance of vital energies (Qi) and the circulation of bodily fluids, may have been influenced by early practices like stove-based bathing.

While the details of stove-based bathing are not extensively documented, archaeological evidence and historical texts suggest that the ancient Chinese had a nuanced understanding of the benefits of heat bathing. The practice of stove-based bathing laid the foundation for the development of more intricate bathing traditions in China and contributed to the broader global history of heat bathing practices.

2. Native American Sweat Lodges:

Native American dry sweat practices, often conducted within a structure known as a sweat lodge, hold deep spiritual, communal, and healing significance. These practices vary among different tribes, but they share common elements centered around purification, prayer, and connection to the spiritual realm. Let's explore these practices in depth:

1. Sweat Lodge Structure:
- **Construction:** Sweat lodges are typically small, dome-shaped structures constructed with a frame of willow or other flexible branches. The frame is covered with blankets, hides, or other materials to create an enclosed space.

- **Symbolism:** The construction of the sweat lodge often involves symbolic elements, representing the womb of Mother Earth. The entrance is seen as a symbolic birth canal.

2. Heating Stones and Creating Steam:

- **Heated Stones:** Large stones, often referred to as "Grandfathers," are heated in an external fire until they become red-hot. Referring to the stones as "grandfathers" is a practice often associated with the Lakota Sioux tribe during their sweat lodge ceremonies. The Lakota people, who are part of the larger Sioux Nation, hold the sweat lodge ceremony, known as the *Inipi* ceremony, in high regard. In the Lakota tradition, the heated stones play a symbolic and revered role, and they are often addressed as "grandfathers" as a sign of respect for their spiritual significance during the ceremony. It's important to note that terminologies and practices can vary among different Native American tribes, and while the use of "grandfathers" specifically aligns with the Lakota tradition, other tribes may have different names or symbolic meanings for the heated stones in their respective sweat lodge ceremonies.

- **Placing Stones:** The heated stones are then carefully brought inside the sweat lodge and placed in a central pit or alter.

3. Ceremonial Process:

- **Purification Ritual:** Participants, or "sweatlodge keepers," engage in a purification ritual before entering the sweat lodge. This may involve smudging with sacred herbs like sage or sweetgrass.

- **Four Rounds:** The sweat lodge ceremony typically consists of four rounds, each with a specific purpose, such as purification, prayer, or seeking guidance.

- **Prayers and Songs:** Participants offer prayers and sing traditional songs, creating a spiritual atmosphere within the lodge.

4. Duration and Intensity:

- **Varied Duration:** The duration of a sweat lodge ceremony can vary among tribes and communities. Some may last a few hours, while others, especially during specific rituals or ceremonies, can extend throughout the night or even several days.

- **Intense Heat:** The heat inside the sweat lodge can be intense, symbolizing the challenges and purification process. Participants endure the heat to connect with the spiritual realm and receive guidance.

5. Spiritual Significance:

- **Connection to Creator:** The sweat lodge is viewed as a sacred space where participants connect with the Creator, Mother Earth, and the spirit world. It's a place for seeking guidance, healing, and spiritual insight.

Purification: The sweat ceremony is seen as a purification process, not just physically but also spiritually and emotionally. It's a way of cleansing oneself of negative energy and seeking balance.

6. Cultural Variations:

- **Diverse Practices:** Different tribes have unique variations of sweat lodge practices. The Lakota, for example, have the *Inipi* ceremony, while the Ojibwe practice the *Baapanjiimowin* ceremony. Each tribe may have specific rituals, songs, and prayers associated with their sweat lodge practices.

7. Contemporary Relevance:

- **Cultural Continuity:** Despite historical challenges, Native American sweat lodge practices continue to be relevant and meaningful for many indigenous communities today. Efforts to preserve and revitalize these traditions are ongoing.

8. Cultural Sensitivity:

- **Respect for Traditions:** When exploring or discussing Native American sweat lodge practices, it's essential to approach the subject with cultural sensitivity, recognizing the sacred nature of these ceremonies and respecting the diversity of tribal traditions.

In essence, Native American dry sweat practices, conducted within sweat lodges, are deeply rooted in spiritual traditions, emphasizing purification, connection with the spiritual realm, and the pursuit of balance and well-being. These practices continue to play a crucial role in many Native American communities, maintaining cultural identity and spirituality.

3. Ancient Greek and Roman Dry Heat:

Ancient Rome is renowned for its elaborate thermal baths, such as the Baths of Caracalla and the Baths of Diocletian. These bathhouses featured rooms with varying temperatures, including hot rooms resembling sauna-like environments. Romans used these baths for socializing, relaxation, and maintaining personal hygiene.

Below is a description of the *caldarium*, *laconicum*, and *sudatorium* in the context of ancient Greek and Roman dry heat therapies:

1. Caldarium:

- **Description:** The *caldarium* was the hot room in a Roman bathhouse, designed to provide intense dry heat.

- **Heating System:** It featured a *hypocaust* system where hot air circulated beneath the floor and walls, creating a consistently heated environment.

- **Temperature:** The *caldarium* maintained a high temperature, often utilizing heated pools and steam to enhance the heat.

- **Purpose:** The intense heat in the *caldarium* was believed to open pores, induce sweating, and promote a sense of relaxation. It also contributed to the overall cleansing process.

2. Laconicum:

- **Description:** The *laconicum* was a room similar to a modern sauna, providing dry heat therapy but typically at a slightly lower temperature than the *caldarium*.

- **Construction:** Similar to the *caldarium*, the *laconicum* used the *hypocaust* system for heating, but the temperature was moderated to create a warm and relaxing environment.

- **Sweating and Detoxification:** The *laconicum* aimed to induce sweating and promote detoxification. The name *"laconicum"* is derived from *Laconia*, the region in ancient Greece known for the Spartan warriors, suggesting a connection to physical fitness and endurance.

3. Sudatorium:

- **Description:** The *sudatorium* was a specialized room designed for sweating and detoxification.

- **Temperature:** Like the *caldarium* and *laconicum*, the *sudatorium* featured elevated temperatures. However, the focus was on creating an environment conducive to perspiration.

- **Purpose:** The *sudatorium* aimed to encourage profuse sweating, believed to cleanse the body of impurities and contribute to overall well-being.

- **Structural Features:** The room often had features to enhance the heating effect, such as alcoves for reclining and strategic placement of hot air vents.

4. Similarities and Purposes:

- **Thermal Sequence:** In Roman bathhouses, these rooms were often arranged in a sequence, with the *frigidarium* (cold room), *tepidarium* (warm room), *caldarium* (hot room), and sometimes the *sudatorium* or *laconicum*, providing a range of temperature experiences.

- **Health and Well-Being:** The use of these heated rooms was associated with various health benefits, including improved circulation, muscle relaxation, and detoxification. They were also places for socializing and relaxation.

5. Influence on Contemporary Practices:

- **Legacy:** The concept of heated rooms in Roman bathhouses has had a lasting impact on contemporary spa and wellness practices, with saunas and similar facilities offering dry heat therapy for relaxation and health benefits.

The *caldarium*, *laconicum*, and *sudatorium* were integral components of ancient Greek and Roman dry heat therapies. Each room provided a unique thermal experience, contributing to the overall bathing ritual and reflecting the cultural importance placed on physical well-being, relaxation, and social interaction in these ancient societies.

4. Mayan Sweat Houses:

The ancient Maya civilization (2000 BCE to 1500 CE) had sweat houses, or *"temazcals,"* used for rituals and healing. These structures were designed for steam ceremonies involving heated stones and herbal infusions, promoting both physical and spiritual well-being.

The Mayan *temazcal* ceremonies typically involve a combination of both dry heat and steam. The structure of the *temazcal* is designed to allow for the heating of stones, and the addition of medicinal herbs to create steam. Participants experience a mix of dry heat from the heated stones and the humidifying effects of the infused steam.

The dry heat comes from the radiant energy of the hot stones within the enclosed space, promoting sweating and aiding in physical purification. The steam, often infused with aromatic herbs, adds another layer to the experience, contributing to the therapeutic and spiritual aspects of the ceremony. The combination of dry heat and steam creates a unique and intense environment within the *temazcal*, symbolizing purification, rebirth, and connection to the elements in Mayan cosmology.

Mayan sweat houses, known as *"temazcals,"* were integral to the cultural and spiritual practices of the ancient Maya civilization. These sweat houses played a crucial role in rituals, healing ceremonies, and community activities. Here is an examination of Mayan sweat houses, including their structure, purpose, cultural significance, and contemporary relevance:

1. Structure of *Temazcals*:
- **Design:** *Temazcals* were typically small, dome-shaped structures made from stone or adobe bricks.

- **Entrance:** The entrance to the *temazcal* represented the birth canal, emphasizing the symbolism of rebirth and purification.

2. Heating Elements:
- **Heated Stones:** Similar to other indigenous sweat lodge practices, the Mayan *temazcal* involved heating stones to produce steam.

- **Herbal Infusions:** Maya shamans often infused the steam with medicinal herbs, adding a therapeutic element to the sweating ritual.

3. Rituals and Ceremonies:
- **Purification:** The primary purpose of the *temazcal* was purification—both physical and spiritual.

- **Connection to the Elements:** Rituals conducted inside the *temazcal* were believed to connect individuals to the four elements: earth, air, water, and fire.

4. Spiritual Significance:
- **Connection to Deities:** Sweating ceremonies in the *temazcal* were often associated with invoking the presence of deities and spirits.

- **Rebirth Symbolism:** The symbolism of the t*emazcal's* structure, resembling a womb, emphasized the theme of rebirth and renewal.

5. Healing Practices:
- **Therapeutic Effects:** The steam and herbal infusions were considered to have therapeutic effects, promoting physical well-being and cleansing the body of impurities.

- **Shamanic Healing:** Shamans played a central role in conducting ceremonies within the *temazcal*, using the environment to facilitate healing and spiritual experiences.

6. Community and Social Aspects:

- **Community Gatherings:** The *temazcal* served as a communal space, bringing people together for shared experiences and rituals.

- **Cultural Identity:** Participation in *temazcal* ceremonies reinforced cultural identity and community bonds among the Maya.

7. Contemporary Practices:

- **Cultural Preservation:** In some modern Maya communities, efforts are made to preserve and revitalize *temazcal* ceremonies as part of cultural heritage.

- **Tourism:** *Temazcal* experiences have also become popular attractions for tourists seeking a traditional Mayan sweat lodge experience.

8. Cultural Sensitivity:

- **Respect for Traditions:** Understanding and respecting the cultural significance of *temazcals* is crucial. Visitors participating in or observing *temazcal* ceremonies should approach these practices with cultural sensitivity.

Mayan sweat houses, through the *temazcal* ceremony, provided the ancient Maya with a sacred space for purification, healing, and spiritual connection. While contemporary practices may vary, efforts to preserve these traditions underscore the enduring cultural significance of the *temazcal* in the Maya community.

5. Ancient Finland:

In Ancient Finland, one of the birthplaces of the modern sauna, early versions were likely primitive smoke saunas. These were simple structures with an open fire, and stones heated by the fire provided warmth. The smoke was then allowed to escape before individuals entered.

1. Construction and Design:
- **Simple Structures:** Primitive smoke saunas were basic and often built with logs, stones, and sod to form a small, enclosed space.

- **Earthen Floor:** The floor of the sauna was typically made of earth or gravel.

2. Heating Method:
- **Wood-Burning Stove:** The heating method in these saunas involved a wood-burning stove, which generated both heat and smoke.

- **Smoke Channels:** The smoke from the burning wood would circulate within the sauna, contributing to the distinctive atmosphere.

3. Ventilation System:
- **Limited Ventilation:** Primitive saunas had limited ventilation, allowing the smoke to permeate the interior. The controlled ventilation helped maintain the right balance of heat and smoke.

4. Usage and Rituals:
- **Daily Practices:** Saunas were an integral part of daily life in ancient Finland. The smoke saunas were used for bathing, relaxation, and various rituals.

- **Cleansing Rituals:** Saunas were places for both physical and spiritual cleansing. Sweating in the heat and the subsequent plunge into cold water or snow was a common practice.

5. Social Aspects:
- **Community Gathering:** Saunas served as communal spaces, providing opportunities for socializing, discussions, and bonding among community members.

- Cultural Significance: The sauna experience was deeply intertwined with Finnish culture and held significant importance in social and family life.

6. Transition to Modern Saunas:
- **Evolution of Sauna Design:** Over time, the design and construction of saunas evolved. The primitive smoke saunas paved the way for more sophisticated sauna structures, including those with improved heating systems and ventilation.

7. Cultural Continuity:
- **Enduring Tradition:** While the technology and design have evolved, the sauna remains an enduring tradition in Finland. Modern saunas still incorporate elements of the ancient smoke saunas, emphasizing the cultural and social aspects of sauna bathing.

8. Cultural Symbolism:
- **Symbolism of Smoke:** The smoke in these primitive saunas was not just a byproduct but held cultural symbolism. It contributed to the ritualistic and sacred nature of the sauna experience, connecting the physical and spiritual realms.

9. Sauna in Finnish Identity:

- **National Symbol:** The sauna has become a national symbol of Finland, reflecting the deep cultural, social, and historical ties that the Finnish people have with this tradition.

Smoke and Safety:

While the smoke in primitive smoke saunas was an inherent part of the heating process, the controlled use of smoke in these saunas was not considered inherently dangerous when managed properly. The construction and design of the saunas were developed to balance the benefits of heat with the presence of smoke. However, it's essential to note a few key points:

1. Ventilation Control: Primitive smoke saunas had limited ventilation, and the control of ventilation was crucial. This allowed for a sufficient amount of smoke to circulate within the sauna, contributing to the unique atmosphere and heat, while preventing an excessive buildup that could be harmful.

2. Cautious Use of Wood: The choice of wood for the stove was essential. Certain types of wood produce less harsh or irritating smoke. Careful selection of wood helped mitigate potential health risks associated with smoke inhalation.

3. Experience and Tradition: Over time, the Finnish people developed an understanding of how to use and manage the smoke in saunas. The experience of sauna-goers and the cultural knowledge passed down through generations contributed to a safe and enjoyable sauna experience.

4. Evolution of Sauna Design: As sauna technology evolved, improvements in ventilation systems and heating methods were introduced, reducing the reliance on smoke for heat. Modern saunas, while still preserving the cultural essence of sauna bathing, incorporate advancements that enhance safety and comfort.

While controlled exposure to smoke in the traditional setting of smoke saunas was generally considered safe within the context of Finnish cultural practices, it's important to recognize that prolonged or excessive exposure to smoke, especially in unventilated spaces, can have health risks. In modern saunas, there is a greater emphasis on proper ventilation, and many saunas use alternative heating methods, such as electric or infrared heaters, to achieve a comfortable and safe sauna experience. Individuals with respiratory conditions or concerns should exercise caution and may want to consult with healthcare professionals before using saunas, especially those with significant smoke exposure.

The primitive smoke saunas in ancient Finland laid the foundation for the rich tradition of sauna bathing in Finnish culture. These early saunas were not only places for physical cleansing but also held social, cultural, and spiritual significance, shaping the sauna practices that continue to thrive in Finland and around the world today.

6. Korean hanjeungmak

The history of Korean *hanjeungmak*, a traditional Korean dry heat sauna, is deeply rooted in the country's bathing culture, reflecting both practical and cultural aspects. Here's an overview of the history of *hanjeungmak*:

1. Ancient Origins:
•   The roots of Korean bathing culture can be traced back to ancient times. Early forms of bathing likely involved natural hot springs and communal bathing practices.

2. Introduction of *Hanjeungmak*:
•   *Hanjeungmak*, as a distinctive dry heat sauna, is thought to have originated during the Goryeo Dynasty (918–1392) or earlier.

•   The term *"hanjeung"* refers to a space heated with fire, and *"mak"* means room, denoting a heated room.

3. Goryeo Dynasty (918–1392):
•   The Goryeo Dynasty played a crucial role in shaping Korean culture and traditions, including bathing practices.

•   Early *hanjeungmak* may have been influenced by similar practices in neighboring East Asian cultures.

4. Joseon Dynasty (1392–1897):
•   The Joseon Dynasty continued and further developed the Korean bathing culture, including *hanjeungmak*.

•   Public bathhouses, including those with *hanjeungmak* facilities, became more common during this period.

5. Construction and Design:
•   Traditional *hanjeungmak* facilities were constructed with materials like wood, stone, and clay, creating a heated environment.

•   The design often featured a series of kiln-like structures to generate heat.

6. Sauna Culture Development:
- Over the centuries, the practice of using *hanjeungmak* evolved, and it became an integral part of Korean sauna culture.

- Different regions in Korea developed their variations of *hanjeungmak*.

7. Bathhouses and Community Spaces:
- *Hanjeungmak* was not only a personal practice but also a communal one. Public bathhouses, where *hanjeungmak* was a central feature, served as important social spaces.

8. Bathhouse Rituals:
- Bathhouses in Korea were not just places for physical cleansing but also spaces for socializing and relaxation.

- Bathhouse rituals included scrubbing, massage, and the use of various herbal treatments.

9. Modern Era and Globalization:
- In the modern era, *hanjeungmak* has adapted to changing lifestyles and technology.

- Today, *hanjeungmak* is not only part of traditional bathhouses but can also be found in modern spa facilities.

10. Health and Wellness:
- *Hanjeungmak* is believed to offer various health benefits, including improved circulation, skin detoxification, and stress relief.

11. Cultural Significance:
- *Hanjeungmak* holds cultural significance in Korea, symbolizing relaxation, cleansing, and a connection to traditional practices.

12. Contemporary *Hanjeungmak* Facilities:
- In contemporary times, *hanjeungmak* facilities often include a variety of heat rooms with different temperatures and features, creating a diverse sauna experience.

While the exact historical origins may not be precisely documented, *hanjeungmak's* long history underscores its enduring importance in Korean bathing culture. The practice continues to thrive, offering both locals and visitors a unique and culturally rich sauna experience in Korea.

6B. Korean Salt Saunas - *Jjimjilbang:*

Korean heated salt rooms, often referred to as "*Jjimjilbang*" or "Salt Saunas," are spaces designed for relaxation and wellness. These rooms typically feature heated walls made of salt and are part of larger spa and sauna complexes known as *Jjimjilbangs* in Korean culture. Here's an overview of Korean heated salt rooms:

Characteristics

1. Salt Walls:
The walls of these rooms are often made of salt bricks or salt crystals. The salt is heated to release negative ions, which are believed to have various health benefits.

2. Heating Element:
The rooms are equipped with a heating element to maintain a warm temperature. The heat enhances the therapeutic effects of the salt and creates a comfortable environment for visitors.

3. Salt Inhalation:
In some salt rooms, there may be mechanisms for salt inhalation. This can include finely ground salt particles in the air, similar to the experience of being near natural salt caves.

4. Color Therapy:
Some salt rooms incorporate color therapy, with different colored lights used to enhance the overall relaxing atmosphere. This may contribute to a sensory and visual experience.

5. Relaxation Seating:
The rooms typically have comfortable seating, allowing visitors to relax and unwind while enjoying the therapeutic effects of the salt.

Health Benefits (Perceived)

1. Respiratory Benefits:
Salt is believed to have anti-inflammatory and antimicrobial properties, potentially benefiting individuals with respiratory issues such as asthma or allergies.

2. Skin Health:
Salt is thought to have positive effects on the skin. The salt particles in the air may contribute to skin exfoliation and improved circulation.

3. Stress Reduction:
The combination of heat, salt, and the overall calming environment is intended to promote relaxation and reduce stress.

4. Detoxification:
Some proponents suggest that the salt sauna experience aids in the detoxification process by helping the body eliminate toxins.

The *Jjimjilbang* Experience

Korean *Jjimjilbangs* are comprehensive wellness complexes that often include various sauna rooms, hot baths, cold baths, relaxation areas, and additional amenities such as restaurants and entertainment facilities. Visitors typically move between different rooms, each offering a unique sauna experience, including the salt rooms.

It's important to note that while many people find these experiences enjoyable and relaxing, scientific evidence supporting specific health claims associated with salt rooms is limited. As with any wellness practice, individual experiences and perceived benefits can vary.

If you're interested in trying a Korean heated salt room, consider visiting a *Jjimjilbang* or a spa that offers these facilities. Always follow the guidelines provided by the facility and consult with healthcare professionals if you have specific health concerns.

These early sauna-like practices were not only about physical cleansing but often held spiritual, social, and cultural significance. The concept of using heat for health and relaxation has deep roots in human history, evolving over time into the diverse sauna traditions we see today. The development of saunas as a distinct cultural and wellness practice continued to flourish in regions like Scandinavia, where it became an integral part of daily life and communal rituals.

3. Nordic Sauna Culture

Nordic sauna culture is deeply rooted in rituals, customs, and social practices that extend beyond mere bathing. It's a dynamic and evolving aspect of Nordic identity, blending tradition with contemporary influences. The sauna is not just a physical space; it's a cultural phenomenon that fosters community, well-being, and a unique sense of Nordic belonging.

1. Rituals and Customs:

A. The Sauna Session:
- **Frequency:** Sauna bathing is a regular and cherished practice in Nordic cultures. It's common for families to have saunas at home, and public saunas are prevalent in communities.

- **Sequential Bathing:** Sauna sessions often follow a specific sequence, starting with time in the sauna, followed by cooling off, and possibly repeating the process.

B. *Aufguss (Löyly)*:
- **Enhancing the Experience:** The practice of *"aufguss"* or *"löyly"* involves throwing water on heated sauna stones to create steam. This ritual is often performed with essential oils, enhancing the aroma and sensory experience.

- **Therapeutic Benefits:** *Aufguss* is not just about heating; it's a performance that adds a therapeutic element to the sauna session, contributing to physical and mental well-being.

C. Sauna Whisk (*Vihta/Vasta*):
- **Birch Whisk Ritual:** The use of sauna whisks, typically made of birch branches, is a tradition. Bathers lightly beat themselves or each other with the *vihta* or *vasta*, promoting circulation and relaxation.

- **Symbolism:** The birch whisk is symbolic of nature's purity and is believed to enhance the sauna experience.

D. Cooling Off in Nature:
- **Nature Integration:** Cooling off between sauna sessions often involves immersion in natural bodies of water, be it a lake, river, or icy plunge pool. This connection with nature is integral to the Nordic sauna experience.

2. Social Importance and Cultural Evolution:

A. Social Gathering Spaces:
- **Family and Community:** Saunas are social spaces. Families gather in saunas at home, and communities have public saunas where people of all ages socialize.

- **Community Sauna Events:** Some communities organize sauna events, fostering a sense of togetherness and cultural identity.

B. Business and Diplomacy:
- **Sauna Diplomacy:** Saunas play a unique role in business and diplomacy. "Sauna diplomacy" refers to informal meetings that take place in saunas, emphasizing openness and equality.

- **Networking and Bonding:** Saunas are often venues for networking and bonding, breaking down hierarchical barriers.

C. Cultural Evolution:
- **Historical Roots:** The roots of Nordic sauna culture extend back centuries, with saunas initially serving practical purposes of bathing and hygiene.

- **Evolution of Sauna Technology:** From traditional wood-burning saunas to modern electric or infrared saunas, technology has evolved, but the cultural significance remains.

D. Sauna Clubs and Societies:
- **Promoting Sauna Culture:** Sauna clubs and societies actively promote sauna culture. These organizations organize events, competitions, and educational programs to engage enthusiasts.

- **Sauna Competitions:** Sauna enthusiasts participate in competitions, testing endurance and heat tolerance.

E. Wellness and Holistic Health:
- **Holistic Well-Being:** Sauna culture is intertwined with notions of holistic health. Regular sauna bathing is viewed as a means of promoting physical, mental, and emotional well-being.

- **Stress Reduction:** Saunas are considered stress-relief sanctuaries, providing an escape from the pressures of daily life.

F. Sauna Architecture:

- **Architectural Diversity:** Sauna architecture ranges from traditional log cabins to contemporary urban designs. Some saunas offer panoramic views, contributing to a unique and immersive experience.

- **Sauna as Art:** In some instances, saunas are designed as art installations, showcasing the fusion of architecture and cultural expression.

G. Global Impact:

- **International Recognition:** Nordic sauna culture has gained international recognition. Sauna practices, events, and designs have influenced global wellness trends.

- **Sauna Tourism:** Sauna tourism is on the rise, with people from around the world seeking authentic Nordic sauna experiences.

§

4. Russian *Banyas* vs Nordic Sauna

The Russian *banya* has a rich historical development deeply intertwined with Russian culture and societal practices. Its role extends beyond mere bathing, encompassing social, cultural, and even spiritual dimensions. Today, the *banya* remains a symbol of communal well-being and a testament to the enduring cultural identity of Russia.

While both the Russian *banya* and the Nordic sauna share similarities as heat bathing traditions, they have distinct origins, cultural contexts, and evolutionary paths. Here's a comparison highlighting the differences:

Origins:

1. Russian Banya:
Roots in Slavic and Finnish Cultures: The Russian banya has roots in both Slavic and Finnish cultures. The term *"banya"* itself has Finnish origins, and early bathing practices in Slavic tribes influenced its development.

Symbolism in Folklore: The *banya* is often symbolically significant in Russian folklore, representing purity, fertility, and health.

2. Nordic Sauna:
Primarily Finnish Origin: The Nordic sauna, particularly the sauna culture prevalent in Finland, has a predominantly Finnish origin.

Ancient Beginnings: The sauna tradition in Finland dates back thousands of years, evolving from simple pit-like structures to the sophisticated saunas seen today.

Evolution:

1. Russian Banya:
- **Social and Cultural Evolution:** The Russian *banya* has evolved as a social and cultural hub, serving as a communal gathering space with deep ties to traditional ceremonies and celebrations.

- **Urbanization and Modernization:** In urban settings, traditional *banyas* have adapted to modern amenities, preserving cultural practices while incorporating contemporary features.

2. Nordic Sauna:
- **Integration into Everyday Life:** The Finnish sauna is deeply integrated into everyday life, with many households having their saunas. Sauna

bathing is a regular practice, and the sauna is considered a place for relaxation and well-being.

- **Global Recognition:** Finnish sauna culture has gained international recognition, influencing wellness practices worldwide. It has become a symbol of Finnish identity and lifestyle.

Cultural Differences:

1. Russian *Banya*:
- **Social Equality Emphasis:** The *banya* is known for breaking down social hierarchies, creating an atmosphere of equality and camaraderie, especially in the heated room (*"parilka"*).

- **Iconic Imagery:** Images of people in *banyas*, surrounded by steam and using *veniks*, are iconic representations of Russian cultural practices.

2. Nordic Sauna:
- **Solo and Family Practices:** While social sauna sessions exist, sauna bathing in Nordic cultures, particularly in Finland, often involves solo or family experiences. It is a time for personal reflection and relaxation.

- **Sauna Diplomacy:** Saunas in Nordic cultures, while still social spaces, may not emphasize the same level of communal equality as seen in Russian *banyas*.

Modern Practices:

1. Russian *Banya*:
- **Preservation of Tradition:** Efforts are made to preserve traditional *banya* practices, ensuring that cultural heritage remains intact.

- **Global Appeal:** *Banyas* have gained international appeal, attracting wellness enthusiasts seeking authentic cultural experiences.

2. Nordic Sauna:
- **Evolution in Urban Settings:** Saunas in urban settings have evolved with modern amenities, offering a blend of tradition and contemporary features.

- **Wellness Tourism:** Finnish sauna practices are sought after globally, contributing to wellness tourism and cultural exchange.

5. Understanding Japanese *Sento* and *Ganban'yoku*

Japanese *sento* and *ganban'yoku* are deeply rooted in the country's rich bathing culture. While *sento* reflects historical communal bathing traditions in urban settings, *ganban'yoku* represents a modern evolution with a focus on dry heat therapy. Both have adapted to contemporary lifestyles, offering diverse experiences that blend tradition with innovation. The cultural significance of bathing in Japan, rooted in cleanliness, purification, and relaxation, continues to thrive and has become a globally recognized aspect of wellness culture.

1. Connection to Japanese Bathing Culture:

A. Historical Roots:
- **Ancient Tradition:** Bathing has deep roots in Japanese culture, dating back to ancient times. Early communal bathing practices were influenced by religious and social customs.

- **Onsen Tradition:** The *onsen*, or hot springs, have been a significant part of Japanese bathing culture. *Onsen* bathing has therapeutic connotations, with mineral-rich waters believed to have health benefits.

B. *Sento*:
- **Urban Bathhouses:** *Sento* refers to public bathhouses found in urban areas. Historically, not all households had access to private baths, making *sento* crucial for communal bathing.

- **Community Spaces:** *Sento* served as social hubs, fostering community interaction. They played a role in maintaining hygiene, especially in densely populated cities.

C. *Ganban'yoku*:
- **Stone Bathing Tradition:** *Ganban'yoku*, or stone bathing, is a more recent addition to Japanese bathing culture. It involves lying on heated stone slabs, often made of black silica or other minerals.

- **Thermal Therapy:** *Ganban'yoku* is rooted in the concept of thermal therapy, with the heated stones providing a dry heat experience that promotes relaxation and wellness.

D. Cultural Significance:

- **Ceremonial Aspects:** Bathing in Japan is often considered a ceremonial act. Before entering a bath, individuals typically wash and rinse thoroughly, emphasizing cleanliness and purification.

- **Symbolism in Shinto:** Bathing has symbolic significance in Shinto rituals, representing spiritual and physical purification.

2. Modern Adaptations:

A. *Sento* in Modern Japan:

- **Evolution in Urban Context:** While traditional *sento* still exists, modern *sento* facilities have adapted to urban lifestyles, offering diverse amenities, entertainment, and relaxation spaces.

- **Art and Design:** Some modern *sento* incorporate art and contemporary design, creating a unique and aesthetically pleasing bathing environment.

- **Wellness Features:** Some *sento* incorporate wellness features such as saunas, Jacuzzis, and relaxation lounges, expanding beyond the traditional bathing experience.

B. *Ganban'yoku* in Contemporary Settings:

- **Wellness Trend:** *Ganban'yoku* has become a wellness trend in Japan and beyond. It is often offered in spa-like settings with additional services like aromatherapy and massage.

- **Themed Facilities:** Some *ganban'yoku* facilities have themed rooms with different types of heated stones, creating a sensory and therapeutic experience.

- **Integration into *Onsen* Resorts:** *Ganban'yoku* experiences are sometimes integrated into *onsen* resorts, offering visitors a combination of traditional hot springs and dry stone bathing.

C. Cultural Preservation:

- **Efforts to Preserve Tradition:** While modern adaptations are present, there are also efforts to preserve the cultural aspects of *sento*. Traditional *sento* with historical significance are sometimes designated as cultural landmarks.

- **Community Events:** Some *sento* host community events, maintaining their role as social hubs where people come together for more than just bathing.

D. Technological Innovation in *Ganban'yoku*:

In the realm of *Ganban'yoku*, or hot stone bathing, technological advances play a pivotal role in enhancing the overall experience for participants. One notable area of innovation lies in the development of advanced heating systems for the stones, enabling a level of precision and customization that transforms the traditional practice.

Traditional *Ganban'yoku* involves the use of heated stones placed on the floor to create a warm and relaxing environment. However, with technological advancements, the heating systems have evolved to offer a more tailored and sophisticated experience. Modern *Ganban'yoku* facilities may employ state-of-the-art equipment that ensures precise temperature control, allowing for a more nuanced and personalized session.

One technological innovation involves the integration of smart heating systems that can be programmed to follow specific temperature profiles throughout the bathing session. This not only caters to individual preferences but also enhances the therapeutic benefits of hot stone bathing. Participants can enjoy a gradual increase or decrease in temperature, creating a dynamic and rejuvenating experience.

Furthermore, advanced heating elements may be embedded within the stones themselves. This eliminates the need for external heat sources, contributing to a more seamless and efficient heating process. These embedded elements can be designed to distribute heat evenly, ensuring that every part of the stone surface reaches the desired temperature. This level of precision enhances the therapeutic effects of *Ganban'yoku*, as the stones can be optimized to release heat in a way that maximizes relaxation and stress relief.

In addition to temperature control, technology has also been integrated into the overall environment of *Ganban'yoku* spaces. Smart lighting, sound systems, and even aromatherapy dispensers can be synchronized to create a multi-sensory experience that complements the soothing effects of hot stone bathing. These innovations allow participants to customize their sessions based on personal preferences, making *Ganban'yoku* a more immersive and enjoyable practice.

Overall, technological advances in *Ganban'yoku* contribute to the evolution of this ancient wellness practice into a modern and highly customizable experience. By incorporating cutting-edge heating systems, smart technology, and other enhancements, *Ganban'yoku* facilities can offer a rejuvenating escape that caters to the diverse preferences of individuals seeking relaxation and therapeutic benefits.

E. Therapeutic Focus: *Ganban'yoku* facilities, with a therapeutic focus, place a strong emphasis on the health and wellness benefits associated with hot stone bathing. By highlighting improvements in circulation, detoxification, and stress reduction, these establishments aim to position *ganban'yoku* as not just a relaxing experience but also a holistic therapeutic practice.

i. Circulation Enhancement:
These facilities often promote the idea that the application of heated stones to the body promotes vasodilation, leading to improved blood circulation. The heat from the stones is believed to cause blood vessels to dilate, facilitating better blood flow to various parts of the body. Improved circulation is associated with benefits such as enhanced oxygen and nutrient delivery to cells, which can contribute to overall well-being.

ii. Detoxification Claims:
Ganban'yoku facilities with a therapeutic focus often assert that the combination of heat and sweating during the bathing session supports the body's natural detoxification processes. Sweating is considered a way for the body to eliminate toxins through the skin. By promoting sweating through the use of heated stones, these facilities suggest that participants can experience a gentle detoxifying effect, ridding the body of impurities.

iii. Stress Reduction Strategies:
The relaxation induced by the heat and the soothing atmosphere in *ganban'yoku* spaces is positioned as an effective stress reduction strategy. The combination of the warm stones, calming ambiance, and often quiet environments creates an ideal setting for participants to unwind and alleviate stress. Stress reduction is not only seen as a psychological benefit but is also believed to have positive effects on physical well-being.

iv. Therapeutic Stone Placement:
These facilities may employ specific techniques in stone placement to target areas of the body associated with tension or discomfort. By strategically positioning the heated stones on key points, practitioners aim to provide localized therapeutic benefits, such as easing muscle tension and promoting relaxation in specific muscle groups.

v. Educational Initiatives:
To reinforce the therapeutic focus, some *ganban'yoku* facilities invest in educational initiatives. This may include providing informational materials, workshops, or consultations with wellness experts to help participants understand the science behind the claimed benefits. By fostering awareness, these facilities aim to empower individuals to make informed decisions about incorporating *ganban'yoku* into their wellness routines.

Ganban'yoku facilities that emphasize therapeutic benefits go beyond promoting the experience as a simple indulgence; they position hot stone bathing as a deliberate practice with potential health-enhancing effects. Whether through improved circulation, detoxification, stress reduction, or targeted stone placement, these facilities aim to provide a comprehensive and scientifically informed approach to the traditional practice of ganban'yoku, appealing to those seeking both relaxation and therapeutic outcomes.

F. Global Influence:
International Appeal: Japanese bathing culture, anchored by the centuries-old traditions of *sento* and *ganban'yoku*, has captivated the global imagination, transcending borders and becoming a focal point in the realm of wellness tourism. The allure of these cultural practices lies in their ability to offer visitors an authentic and immersive encounter with Japan's rich heritage. *Sento,* with its communal bathing rituals, and *ganban'yoku*, with its therapeutic use of heated stones, provide a genuine glimpse into Japanese daily life, fostering cultural exchange and a deeper understanding of local customs among international tourists.

The rise of wellness tourism, characterized by a global pursuit of experiences that promote health and well-being, has played a pivotal role in the international appeal of Japanese bathing culture. *Sento* and *ganban'yoku* align seamlessly with the principles of holistic wellness, offering relaxation, stress reduction, and potential health benefits. In a world where individuals seek rejuvenation on both physical and mental fronts, these traditional practices resonate strongly with those looking for transformative and meaningful travel experiences.

Educational initiatives within Japanese bathing facilities further enhance the cultural exchange between tourists and the host culture. Visitors actively participate in rituals that have been passed down through generations, gaining insights into the historical and cultural significance of these practices. This not only enriches the travel experience but also fosters a connection between tourists and the destinations they explore.

The visual and experiential nature of Japanese bathing culture makes it highly shareable on social media platforms, where travel influencers and bloggers play a pivotal role in showcasing the serene environments, unique rituals, and aesthetic appeal of *sento* and *ganban'yoku*. This exposure contributes to the international fascination with Japanese bathing culture, enticing a global audience to seek out these authentic experiences.

Recognizing the allure of their bathing culture, Japanese destinations actively market *sento* and *ganban'yoku* experiences to international audiences. These marketing efforts highlight the cultural richness and health benefits associated with traditional Japanese bathing, positioning it as a must-try activity for travelers seeking meaningful and transformative experiences.

The global appeal of Japanese bathing culture, represented by *sento* and *ganban'yoku,* is a harmonious blend of authentic cultural experiences, alignment with wellness tourism trends, educational initiatives, a focus on holistic well-being, social media visibility, and effective destination marketing. As travelers increasingly prioritize meaningful and transformative experiences, Japan's bathing culture stands poised to continue enriching the global tapestry of wellness tourism, offering a unique and rejuvenating perspective on traditional practices in a modern world.

Cultural Exchange: The burgeoning popularity of Japanese bathing practices has initiated a profound cultural exchange, transcending geographical boundaries and encouraging wellness enthusiasts globally to incorporate distinct elements of Japanese bathing into their daily routines. As the allure of sento and ganban'yoku spreads, a growing number of individuals are recognizing the profound impact these practices can have on overall well-being, prompting a cross-cultural adoption of Japanese bathing traditions.

Wellness enthusiasts from diverse corners of the world are increasingly integrating the principles of Japanese bathing into their routines, drawn not only to the physical benefits but also to the holistic and meditative aspects embedded in these age-old practices. The emphasis on relaxation, stress reduction, and the therapeutic use of natural elements, such as hot stones, has resonated strongly with individuals seeking a more mindful and rejuvenating approach to self-care.

Moreover, the global embrace of Japanese bathing culture extends beyond the confines of private homes and personal practices. Wellness retreats, spas, and fitness centers worldwide are incorporating Japanese-inspired bathing experiences into their offerings, recognizing the universal appeal of these time-honored traditions. This cultural exchange is fostering a mutual appreciation for diverse wellness practices and contributing to a broader conversation about the interconnectedness of global well-being.

As a result, the influence of Japanese bathing practices is becoming increasingly pervasive in the broader landscape of wellness. From innovative spa treatments to wellness retreats that draw inspiration from the serene ambiance of traditional Japanese baths, the global wellness community is acknowledging and integrating the wisdom embedded in Japanese bathing practices. This cultural exchange not only enriches individual self-care routines but also fosters a global dialogue on the diverse approaches to well-being, creating a shared appreciation for the significance of intentional, holistic practices in the pursuit of a balanced and healthy lifestyle.

6. Saunas: Health and Wellness Overview

Saunas in modern times have become integral to health and wellness trends, offering a range of physical and mental benefits. From enhanced circulation and muscle relaxation to stress reduction and improved sleep quality, saunas play a multifaceted role in promoting overall well-being. The integration of saunas into contemporary wellness practices reflects their enduring appeal and adaptability to evolving lifestyles. As scientific research continues to explore the health benefits of sauna bathing, these practices are likely to remain central to holistic approaches to health and wellness.

A. Health and Wellness Trends:

1. Claimed Physical Benefits of Sauna

A. Enhanced Circulation:
- **Increased Blood Flow:** Sauna bathing induces vasodilation, expanding blood vessels and improving circulation. This can lead to increased oxygen delivery to muscles and tissues.

- **Cardiovascular Benefits:** Regular sauna use is associated with cardiovascular improvements, including reduced blood pressure and enhanced heart function.

B. Muscle Relaxation and Recovery:
- **Relief from Tension:** The heat from saunas helps relax muscles, reducing tension and promoting flexibility.

- **Post-Exercise Recovery:** Athletes use saunas to aid in post-exercise recovery, as the heat can alleviate muscle soreness and improve overall recovery time.

C. Detoxification:
- **Sweating Mechanism:** Sauna-induced sweating is a natural detoxification process, eliminating toxins and heavy metals from the body.

- **Skin Purification:** Sweating also cleanses the skin, promoting a healthier complexion.

D. Weight Management:

- **Caloric Expenditure:** Sauna sessions can lead to increased heart rate and calorie expenditure, contributing to weight management efforts.

- **Water Weight Loss:** While sauna-induced weight loss is primarily water weight, it can be beneficial for temporary weight management.

§

2. Claimed Mental Health Benefits of Sauna

A. Stress Reduction & Cortisol Regulation: Sauna bathing, through its heat stress response, is linked to the regulation of cortisol levels. The controlled elevation and subsequent adaptation to heat stress contribute to reduced cortisol release during sauna sessions. The relaxation response triggered by sauna bathing extends beyond the immediate experience, promoting a sense of calm and stress reduction. This holistic approach to stress management is one of the many ways in which saunas contribute to overall well-being and mental health. As research in this field progresses, a deeper understanding of the physiological and psychological effects of sauna bathing on stress regulation will likely emerge. here is an overview of the subject based on studies presented up to 2024.

Sauna Bathing and Cortisol Regulation:

i. Mechanism of Cortisol Release:
- **Normal Stress Response:** Cortisol is a hormone released by the adrenal glands in response to stress. This "fight or flight" hormone prepares the body for a rapid response to a perceived threat.

- **Chronic Stress:** Prolonged exposure to stressors can lead to elevated and sustained cortisol levels, contributing to various health issues, including anxiety, depression, and sleep disturbances.

ii. Sauna-Induced Heat Stress:
- **Heat Stress Response:** Sauna bathing induces a controlled form of stress on the body, known as heat stress.

- **Temperature Elevation:** The elevated temperature in a sauna triggers physiological responses, including increased heart rate and blood flow, to dissipate heat.

iii. Hormonal Response to Sauna Bathing:
- **Endocrine System Activation:** Sauna-induced heat stress activates the endocrine system, including the release of hormones.

- **Cortisol Release:** While cortisol levels initially rise in response to heat stress, the overall effect is a controlled release that is different from the prolonged elevation seen in chronic stress.

iv. Adaptation and Habituation:
- **Acclimatization:** Regular sauna use can lead to the body's acclimatization and habituation to heat stress.

- **Reduced Cortisol Response:** Over time, the body becomes more efficient at handling heat stress, leading to a reduced cortisol response during sauna sessions.

v. Stress Reduction and Psychological Effects:
- **Relaxation Response:** The heat and sensory experience in saunas trigger a relaxation response, activating the parasympathetic nervous system.

- **Lowered Cortisol Levels:** This relaxation response is associated with lowered cortisol levels, contributing to a sense of calm and reduced stress.

vi. Time-Dependent Effects:
- **Post-Sauna Period:** The reduction in cortisol levels may extend beyond the immediate post-sauna period, contributing to sustained stress reduction.

- **Cumulative Benefits:** Regular sauna bathing, as part of a wellness routine, may contribute to cumulative stress reduction over time.

vii. Research Findings:
- **Scientific Studies:** Scientific research on sauna bathing has explored its impact on cortisol levels.

- **Positive Correlation:** Studies suggest a positive correlation between sauna use and the regulation of cortisol, indicating a potential role in stress reduction.

viii. Holistic Wellness Impact:
- **Comprehensive Wellness:** The cortisol-regulating effects of sauna bathing contribute to the holistic wellness impact of sauna use.

- **Mental Health Benefits:** Beyond cortisol regulation, saunas offer mental health benefits, including mood enhancement and improved sleep, further contributing to stress reduction.

ix. Relaxation Response:
*   The heat and sensory experience in saunas trigger a relaxation response, promoting mental well-being. The scientific basis for the statement lies in the intricate interplay of physiological and psychological responses to heat stress and sensory experiences during sauna bathing. The activation of the parasympathetic nervous system, the release of endorphins, modulation of neurotransmitters, and long-term adaptations collectively contribute to a relaxation response and promote mental well-being. The holistic impact of sauna bathing on both the body and mind underscores its role as a therapeutic and wellness practice

§

B. Improved Sleep Quality:
*   **Regulation of Sleep Hormones:** Sauna use, especially in the evening, can aid in the regulation of sleep hormones such as melatonin.

*   **Enhanced Sleep Patterns:** Saunas contribute to a sense of relaxation, potentially improving sleep quality and patterns.

§

C. Mood Enhancement & Endorphin Release: Endorphin release is intricately linked to mental wellbeing, contributing to mood enhancement, stress reduction, and the overall sense of well-being. While physical exercise is a well-established method for inducing endorphin release, sauna bathing, through its heat-induced stress response, offers another avenue for experiencing these mood-enhancing effects. Engaging in activities that promote endorphin release, as part of a broader mental health strategy, can contribute to a positive and resilient mindset. Below are some highlights from study in this area up to 2024.

Endorphin Release and Mental Wellbeing:

1. What Are Endorphins?

A. Natural Painkillers:
*   **Definition:** Endorphins are neurotransmitters produced by the body, often referred to as "feel-good" chemicals.

*   **Natural Pain Relief:** Endorphins act as natural painkillers, helping to alleviate discomfort and reduce the perception of pain.

2. How Endorphins Are Released?

A. Exercise and Physical Activity:
- **Runner's High:** Endorphin release is commonly associated with physical activities, particularly aerobic exercises like running. The "runner's high" is a well-known example.

- **Intensity Matters:** The intensity of exercise is a key factor in triggering endorphin release.

B. Sauna Bathing and Heat Stress:
- **Heat-Induced Release:** Sauna bathing induces heat stress, leading to the production and release of endorphins.

- **Temperature and Duration:** The elevated temperature in saunas, especially during longer sessions, contributes to the endorphin-releasing effect.

C. Painful Stimuli and Stress:
- **Response to Stress and Pain:** Endorphins are released in response to various stressors and painful stimuli.

- **Adaptive Response:** The release of endorphins is considered an adaptive response, helping the body cope with stress and discomfort.

3. The Connection to Mental Wellbeing:

A. Mood Enhancement:
- **Euphoric Effects:** Endorphins create a sense of euphoria and well-being, contributing to improved mood.

- **Reduction in Anxiety:** The mood-enhancing effects of endorphins can help reduce feelings of anxiety.

B. Stress Reduction:
- **Cortisol Regulation:** Endorphins, in conjunction with other neurochemicals, contribute to the regulation of cortisol, the stress hormone.

- **Alleviating Stress Symptoms:** By regulating stress hormones, endorphins play a role in alleviating symptoms associated with stress.

C. Pleasure and Reward Pathways: The regular use of saunas has long been associated with a range of health benefits, both physical and mental. Beyond its apparent effects on relaxation and stress reduction, the practice of sauna bathing is intertwined with the intricate workings of the dopaminergic system. This essay explores the role of endorphins in activating the brain's pleasure and reward pathways and how this phenomenon contributes to the positive reinforcement associated with regular sauna use.

§

Dopaminergic System and Endorphins:
The dopaminergic system, a complex network of neurons in the brain, is intricately involved in the experience of pleasure and reward. Endorphins, the body's natural painkillers, act as neurotransmitters that bind to opioid receptors within this system. In the context of sauna bathing, the elevation of body temperature prompts the release of endorphins, setting in motion a cascade of neurochemical events that activate the dopaminergic system.

Positive Reinforcement Mechanism:
The activation of the dopaminergic system through the release of endorphins creates a positive reinforcement mechanism during sauna sessions. The heightened heat stress triggers the body's natural response to release endorphins, activating the brain's pleasure and reward pathways. This positive reinforcement establishes a link between the sauna experience and feelings of reward and satisfaction, fostering a desire to repeat the activity.

Promoting Relaxation and Stress Reduction:
Regular sauna use serves as a steadfast ally in promoting relaxation and stress reduction, weaving a tapestry of tranquility through consistent stimulation of endorphin release. The sauna, with its enveloping warmth and ritualistic ambiance, becomes a sanctuary where the soothing effects of endorphins orchestrate a symphony of pleasure and relaxation.

The reliability of this endorphin-induced pleasure transforms the sauna into a haven, a refuge from the ceaseless demands and stresses of daily life. As the heat permeates the body and the mind, a gradual unwinding occurs, releasing the tension held within. The sauna session becomes a therapeutic interlude, a pause amidst the hustle and bustle, offering a respite where stress dissipates like wisps of steam.

Positive reinforcement, intricately linked with the pleasure derived from endorphin release, becomes the cornerstone of this stress-reducing ritual. The mind, conditioned by the consistent interplay of heat and hormonal joy, starts to associate the sauna with a profound sense of well-being. The habitual recurrence of this positive reinforcement establishes a comforting routine—a rhythm of relaxation in sync with the steady rise of endorphins.

Over time, individuals forge a symbiotic relationship with their sauna sessions, cultivating a habitual association between the warm embrace of the sauna and a deep-seated sense of mental and emotional balance. The sauna, once a simple wooden chamber, metamorphoses into a holistic retreat, a therapeutic space where the relentless waves of stress are gently lapped away by the soothing waters of endorphin-induced relaxation.

In the mosaic of daily life, where stress is an omnipresent companion, the regularity of sauna use emerges as a beacon of serenity. It is not merely a physical experience but a mental and emotional voyage—a deliberate and mindful choice to recalibrate, to release, and to rejuvenate amidst the comforting radiance of the sauna. Through the consistent elevation of endorphins, the sauna becomes more than a structure; it becomes an intimate accomplice in the ongoing pursuit of peace and well-being.

Enhancing Mood and Mental Well-Being:
The impact of the dopaminergic system on the sauna experience extends beyond physical sensations to mental well-being. The release of endorphins and the subsequent activation of the reward pathways are linked to an improved mood, reduced anxiety, and an overall sense of contentment. As such, regular sauna use becomes a holistic practice that positively influences both physical and mental aspects of well-being.

Long-Term Benefits and Habit Formation:
The consistent activation of the dopaminergic system through endorphin release creates a positive feedback loop that contributes to habit formation. Individuals who incorporate regular sauna sessions into their routine may develop a positive association between the activity and feelings of reward and satisfaction. This reinforcement fosters a sustainable habit, with the neurobiological processes supporting the long-term integration of sauna use into one's lifestyle.

The interplay between the dopaminergic system, endorphin release, and positive reinforcement sheds light on the multifaceted pleasures of sauna bathing. Beyond its immediate effects on relaxation, the neurobiological underpinnings of the sauna experience highlight its profound impact on mental well-being and the formation of positive wellness habits. Understanding the intricacies of these processes invites us to appreciate sauna use not only as a physical practice but as a holistic and neurobiologically significant ritual that contributes to a balanced and fulfilling life.

7. Saunas, Cognitive Function & Reduced Risk of Neurodegenerative Diseases

Regular sauna bathing is associated with several mechanisms that may contribute to a reduced risk of cognitive decline and neurodegenerative diseases. These mechanisms include improved blood flow, neuroprotective effects, enhanced cognitive function, stress reduction, cardiovascular benefits, and anti-inflammatory effects. While the association is promising, ongoing research is crucial to better understand the specific causal relationships and to identify optimal sauna usage patterns for maximizing cognitive health benefits. Additionally, a holistic approach to cognitive health, including factors like diet, physical activity, and mental stimulation, should be considered in conjunction with sauna use for comprehensive brain health.

The statement "Regular sauna bathing has been associated with a reduced risk of cognitive decline and neurodegenerative diseases" suggests a potential link between consistent sauna use and cognitive health. Let's get a bit more tchnical and explore the key factors that contribute to this association:

1. Heat Stress and Neuroprotection:

a. Increased Blood Flow and Oxygenation:
- **Mechanism:** Sauna bathing induces heat stress, leading to vasodilation and increased blood flow.

- **Effect:** Improved blood flow enhances oxygen delivery to the brain, supporting overall brain health and potentially mitigating factors contributing to cognitive decline.

b. Neuroprotective Effects:
- **Heat Shock Proteins:** Sauna-induced heat stress triggers the production of heat shock proteins.

- **Neuroprotection:** Heat shock proteins have neuroprotective effects, helping protect neurons from damage and supporting their survival.

2. Impact on Cognitive Function:

a. Enhanced Neuroplasticity:
- **BDNF Release:** Sauna use has been linked to increased levels of brain-derived neurotrophic factor (BDNF).

- **Neuroplasticity:** BDNF promotes neuroplasticity, the brain's ability to adapt and reorganize, which is crucial for maintaining cognitive function.

b. Improved Learning and Memory:
- **Synaptic Plasticity:** BDNF supports synaptic plasticity, enhancing the strength and adaptability of synaptic connections.

- **Cognitive Benefits:** Enhanced synaptic plasticity is associated with improved learning and memory, reducing the risk of cognitive decline.

3. Stress Reduction and Cortisol Regulation:

a. Reduced Chronic Stress:
- **Stress Response Regulation:** Sauna bathing has been linked to the regulation of cortisol, the stress hormone.

- **Effect:** By reducing chronic stress and cortisol levels, sauna use may contribute to a lower risk of cognitive decline associated with chronic stress.

4. Cardiovascular Health:

a. Impact on Vascular Function:
- **Improved Blood Vessel Function:** Sauna bathing is associated with improved vascular function.

- **Effect:** Enhanced vascular health supports blood flow to the brain, reducing the risk of vascular-related cognitive decline.

b. Reduced Hypertension Risk:
- **Lower Blood Pressure:** Regular sauna use has been linked to reductions in blood pressure.

- **Cognitive Benefits:** Lowering the risk of hypertension is associated with a reduced risk of cognitive decline and neurodegenerative diseases.

5. Anti-Inflammatory Effects:

a. Inflammation and Cognitive Health:
- **Reduced Inflammation:** Sauna bathing has anti-inflammatory effects.

- **Effect:** Chronic inflammation is implicated in neurodegenerative diseases, and reducing inflammation may contribute to a lower risk of cognitive decline.

6. Social and Psychological Factors:

a. Stress Reduction and Mental Wellbeing:
Community and Relaxation: Saunas often serve as communal spaces, promoting social interaction and relaxation.

Psychosocial Impact: Positive psychosocial factors and reduced stress can contribute to better mental health, potentially influencing cognitive function.

7. Considerations and Future Research:

a. Individual Variances:
Response Differences: Individual responses to sauna bathing may vary based on factors such as genetics, overall health, and lifestyle.

Long-Term Studies: More longitudinal studies are needed to establish a clearer understanding of the long-term effects of regular sauna use on cognitive health.

Summary:

Regular sauna bathing is associated with several mechanisms that may contribute to a reduced risk of cognitive decline and neurodegenerative diseases. These mechanisms include improved blood flow, neuroprotective effects, enhanced cognitive function, stress reduction, cardiovascular benefits, and anti-inflammatory effects. While the association is promising, ongoing research is crucial to better understand the specific causal relationships and to identify optimal sauna usage patterns for maximizing cognitive health benefits. Additionally, a holistic approach to cognitive health, including factors like diet, physical activity, and mental stimulation, should be considered in conjunction with sauna use for comprehensive brain health.

§

8. What is BDNF (Brain-Derived Neurotrophic Factor) and How Does It Relate to Sauna?

Sauna use may increase BDNF levels, and the subsequent impact on cognitive function and mental clarity is linked to BDNF's role in supporting neuroplasticity, learning, memory, and mood regulation. The complex interplay between heat stress, physical activity, and metabolic changes during sauna bathing contributes to the release of BDNF, potentially offering cognitive benefits and promoting mental wellbeing.

Let's delve into the explanation of the statement: "Sauna use may increase BDNF levels, which is linked to cognitive function and mental clarity."

1. Brain-Derived Neurotrophic Factor (BDNF)

A. What is BDNF?
- **Definition:** BDNF is a protein that belongs to the neurotrophin family, playing a crucial role in the growth, development, and maintenance of neurons in the brain.

- **Neurotrophins:** Neurotrophins are a family of proteins that support the survival, growth, and differentiation of both developing and mature neurons.

B. BDNF and Neuronal Health:
- **Neuroplasticity:** BDNF is essential for neuroplasticity, which refers to the brain's ability to reorganize itself by forming new neural connections throughout life.

- **Neuron Survival:** BDNF promotes the survival of existing neurons and the growth and differentiation of new neurons and synapses.

2. Role of BDNF in Cognitive Function

A. Cognitive Function and Learning:
- **Neurogenesis:** BDNF supports neurogenesis, the process of generating new neurons in the brain.

- **Synaptic Plasticity:** BDNF enhances synaptic plasticity, which is critical for learning and memory.

B. Mood Regulation:

- **Impact on Mood Disorders:** BDNF is implicated in mood disorders such as depression and anxiety. Low levels of BDNF are associated with these conditions.

- **Antidepressant Effects:** Increasing BDNF levels is considered beneficial for its potential antidepressant effects.

3. How Sauna Use May Increase BDNF Levels:

A. Heat Stress and BDNF Release:

- **Mechanism:** Sauna bathing induces heat stress on the body.

- **BDNF Release:** Heat stress has been linked to the release of BDNF in the brain, possibly as a protective response.

B. Exercise and BDNF Release:

- **Exercise as a Comparable Stimulus:** Sauna use, especially when associated with physical activity like moderate exercise, can contribute to BDNF release.

- **Cross-Stimulus Effects:** Heat stress-induced by saunas may have cross-stimulus effects similar to those observed during physical exercise.

C. Vascular and Metabolic Effects:

- **Improved Blood Flow:** Sauna use is associated with improved blood flow and vascular function.

- **Metabolic Impact:** The metabolic changes induced by sauna bathing may contribute to the release of BDNF.

4. Cognitive Benefits of Increased BDNF:

A. Enhanced Learning and Memory:

The intricate dance between Brain-Derived Neurotrophic Factor (BDNF) and cognitive function reveals a fascinating nexus where neurobiology meets the intricacies of learning and memory. At the core of this relationship lies the concept of synaptic plasticity—the dynamic ability of synapses to adapt and change over time. BDNF, a neurotrophic factor crucial for neuronal survival and function, emerges as a linchpin in orchestrating the cognitive benefits associated with increased synaptic plasticity.

Synaptic plasticity, under the influence of BDNF, transforms the landscape of neural connections. It accomplishes this by fostering the growth and branching of dendrites, the receivers of signals between neurons. The result is a reinforcement of synaptic connections, enhancing their strength and adaptability. BDNF's impact extends further to the fundamental mechanism of Long-Term Potentiation (LTP), a process integral to the formation of lasting memories and the learning of new information.

Moreover, BDNF's influence is not confined to pre-existing synaptic connections. It extends to the realm of neurogenesis, the birth of new neurons. This multifaceted role of BDNF ensures not only the consolidation of existing memories but also the creation of new opportunities for synaptic plasticity, thereby enriching the neural landscape with the potential for fresh learning experiences.

The adaptability of neural circuits, under the guidance of BDNF, becomes a hallmark of cognitive resilience. This adaptability is indispensable for a myriad of cognitive processes, from spatial learning to the flexible integration of novel information into existing neural networks. BDNF's neuroprotective effects add another layer to its cognitive prowess, safeguarding neurons from damage and contributing to their sustained health—a critical factor in the preservation of cognitive abilities, particularly in the context of aging.

As we unravel the intricate interplay between BDNF and synaptic plasticity, we unearth promising implications for cognitive enhancement. Strategies that boost BDNF release or mimic its effects emerge as potential interventions to enhance learning and memory. From educational contexts to therapeutic approaches for cognitive disorders, the understanding of BDNF's role in synaptic plasticity opens avenues for innovative and targeted cognitive interventions.

In conclusion, the cognitive benefits of increased BDNF are intricately woven into the tapestry of synaptic plasticity. Through its modulation of synaptic connections, BDNF creates an environment conducive to optimal learning and memory. This neurobiological symphony invites us to explore the potential of BDNF-centric interventions for cognitive enhancement, offering a glimpse into the fascinating intersection of neuroscience and cognitive well-being.

Elevated levels of Brain-Derived Neurotrophic Factor (BDNF) intricately weave a tale of cognitive enhancement, specifically in the realms of learning processes and memory formation. BDNF emerges as a central protagonist in this neurobiological narrative, steering the course toward improved cognitive function with a spotlight on synaptic plasticity and Long-Term Potentiation (LTP).

At the heart of this cognitive transformation lies BDNF's profound influence on synaptic plasticity. The heightened BDNF levels act as a catalyst, fostering a dynamic environment where neural connections become more adaptable and resilient. This enhancement in synaptic plasticity becomes a key element in the cognitive journey, enabling the brain to refine its responses to stimuli and create an optimal setting for enhanced learning processes.

The narrative deepens as we explore the intricate link between BDNF and LTP—a process synonymous with the consolidation of memories. Elevated BDNF levels orchestrate a harmonious dance with LTP, promoting the strength and persistence of synaptic connections. In this symbiotic relationship, BDNF becomes a guiding force, ensuring that the cellular processes associated with learning and memory are not only activated but also sustained, resulting in a more robust encoding and retrieval of information.

This cognitive odyssey extends to the concept of neurogenesis, where BDNF's influence sparks the birth of new neurons. These freshly minted neurons integrate seamlessly into existing neural networks, expanding the cognitive canvas and providing additional avenues for learning and memory formation. The link between increased BDNF levels and the creation of new neurons becomes a pivotal chapter in the narrative, illustrating the neurobiological mechanisms that contribute to an enriched cognitive landscape.

In essence, the elevation of BDNF emerges as a catalyst for cognitive alchemy, shaping an environment conducive to improved learning processes and memory formation. The intricate interplay between BDNF and synaptic plasticity, LTP, and neurogenesis becomes a symphony of neurobiological events that underpins our ability to adapt, learn, and remember. As we delve into this narrative, we unravel the intricate dance of BDNF, highlighting its role as a key player in the orchestration of cognitive well-being and the enhancement of our fundamental capacities for learning and memory.

B. Neuroprotective Effects:

At the forefront of BDNF's protective embrace is its role in promoting neuronal survival. Acting as a molecular shield, BDNF fortifies existing neurons, fostering an environment where they can thrive and resist damage. This neuroprotective quality is akin to a vigilant guardian ensuring the preservation of the intricate neural architecture, safeguarding against the threats posed by stressors, toxins, and the wear and tear of time.

The significance of BDNF extends beyond the immediate sheltering of neurons; it becomes a beacon of hope against the inevitable march of age-related cognitive decline. Research illuminates a compelling link between higher BDNF levels and a reduced risk of cognitive deterioration associated with aging. This resilience against cognitive decline is akin to a protective cloak woven by BDNF, shielding the mind from the erosive effects of time and enhancing its ability to withstand the challenges posed by advancing years.

As a neurotrophic factor, BDNF not only nurtures the survival of neurons but also fosters their adaptability. Neurons equipped with optimal BDNF support become more resilient, better equipped to navigate the intricate dance of synaptic connections, and adept at maintaining cognitive function despite the natural wear and tear of aging. The neuroprotective effects of BDNF, therefore, extend beyond immediate preservation to cultivate a foundation for sustained cognitive vitality.

In the holistic narrative of brain health, BDNF emerges as a guardian of cognitive resilience, offering a two-fold protection by promoting neuronal survival and fortifying the mind against age-related cognitive decline. The neuroprotective symphony conducted by BDNF paints a hopeful picture—a canvas where the delicate intricacies of the brain are shielded, allowing for not only the longevity of neuronal existence but also the preservation of cognitive acuity in the face of the passage of time.

C. Mental Clarity and Cognitive Function:

BDNF's role in synaptic plasticity is particularly crucial. The enhancement of synaptic plasticity by BDNF ensures that neural connections remain flexible and adaptable, allowing individuals to grasp new concepts, retain information, and engage in continuous learning. The symbiotic relationship between BDNF and synaptic plasticity creates a neurobiological landscape where the mind is not only agile and receptive but also equipped with the tools for continuous learning and enhanced cognitive performance.

BDNF is emerging as the guardian of cognitive brilliance, navigating the delicate balance between optimal brain function and mental clarity. The science-backed association between increased BDNF levels and mental clarity unveils a pathway towards unlocking the full potential of cognitive brilliance—a journey where the symphony of neurobiological processes harmonizes to elevate cognitive function and illuminate the path to sustained mental acuity.

5. Considerations and Future Research:

A. Individual Variability:
- **Response Differences:** Individuals may show variability in their response to stimuli that increase BDNF levels.

- **Genetic Factors:** Genetic factors can influence an individual's baseline BDNF levels and response to stimuli.

B. Holistic Cognitive Health:
- **Multifaceted Approach:** While BDNF is a key player, cognitive health is i nfluenced by various factors, including nutrition, sleep, and overall lifestyle.

- **Comprehensive Wellbeing:** A holistic approach to cognitive health involves addressing multiple aspects of lifestyle and health.

9. The Sacred Art of Sauna: A Journey of Connection and Well-Being

In the mosaic of human existence, cultural and personal rituals form the vibrant threads that weave a tapestry of identity, community, and well-being. The sauna, a timeless sanctuary of warmth and rejuvenation, emerges as a sacred space where these threads intertwine, contributing to a holistic sense of ritualistic and cultural identity. As we embark on this exploration of the profound significance of saunas in cultural and personal rituals, we delve into the heart of human experience, where intentional practices foster a sense of balance, connection to oneself and others, and a deep-rooted connection to cultural traditions.

Cultural and personal rituals, intrinsic to the human experience, play an indispensable role in shaping our identity and fostering a sense of belonging. They are threads that connect us to our cultural heritage, provide stability in the face of life's flux, and offer an emotional canvas for expression. Sauna bathing, deeply embedded in cultural traditions, becomes a poignant expression of these rituals, carrying the weight of generational continuity and cultural significance.

In the tapestry of rituals, the importance of identity and connection unfolds as a narrative of cultural richness. Rituals, whether shared within a community or observed individually, become a bridge to the past, a vessel that carries the essence of cultural identity. Sauna bathing, with its deep cultural roots, becomes a vessel through which individuals connect not only with their heritage but also with the collective experiences of their community.

Emotional significance weaves another layer into the fabric of rituals, where personal meaning intertwines with symbolic expression. Sauna rituals, marking milestones, transitions, and moments of reflection, offer individuals a structured and symbolic outlet for expressing and processing emotions. The comforting embrace of routine and stability provided by rituals becomes particularly pronounced in the sauna, a place where the predictability of the ritual provides a sense of comfort and security in an ever-changing world.

Mindfulness and reflection, intrinsic to many rituals, become a meditative dance in the sauna's heat and steam. The intentional practice of sauna bathing requires focused attention, promoting mindfulness and being present in the moment. Through this mindful engagement, individuals not only attend to the sensations of heat and relaxation but also reflect on their values, beliefs, and experiences, contributing to a deeper understanding of self.

In the sacred realm of saunas, where cultural and personal rituals converge, the role of this wellness practice becomes profoundly apparent. Sauna bathing is not merely a physical activity but a ritualistic celebration of cultural traditions, community bonds, and personal well-being. It transcends the ordinary, offering a sanctuary for spiritual connection and a means for individuals to connect with something greater than themselves.

Sauna rituals, deeply integrated into cultural practices, hold significance not only in communal settings but also in personal wellness routines. The communal sessions of sauna bathing foster social interaction, strengthen community bonds, and provide shared experiences that enhance social cohesion. Simultaneously, the solitary nature of sauna bathing offers individuals a private space for personal reflection and contemplation, contributing to personal growth and self-awareness.

As we navigate the landscape of sauna rituals, we encounter their integration into daily life—a daily or weekly practice that contributes to a sense of structure and consistency. The sauna becomes a daily wellness ritual, prioritizing and maintaining personal well-being as individuals immerse themselves in the cleansing heat and the mindful embrace of solitude.

The sauna stands as a testament to the enduring significance of cultural and personal rituals in the human experience. As we step into this sacred space, we embark on a journey of connection, well-being, and self-discovery. The sauna's warmth becomes a metaphor for the warmth of cultural identity, the heat of shared experiences, and the steam that clears the path for mental clarity. It is in this sanctuary that the art of sauna bathing unfolds—a timeless expression of the human spirit seeking balance, connection, and the profound beauty of ritual.

10. Sauna Etiquette

is an essential aspect of enjoying the sauna experience, promoting comfort, relaxation, and respect for others.

Following these sauna etiquette and respectful practices ensures that everyone can enjoy the sauna experience in a comfortable and considerate environment. Remember that each sauna setting may have its own specific rules, so always be attentive to posted guidelines and respect the cultural norms of the sauna you are using.

Here's a comprehensive guide to general sauna etiquette and respectful practices:

Before Entering the Sauna:

1. Shower First:
- Always take a thorough shower before entering the sauna. Clean skin promotes a more hygienic sauna experience.

2. Remove Makeup and Lotions:
- Remove makeup and any lotions or oils before entering the sauna. These substances can interact with the heat and affect the sauna's environment.

3. Bring a Towel:
- Always bring a clean towel to sit on. This helps maintain cleanliness and prevents direct contact with the sauna bench.

Inside the Sauna:

4. Choose Appropriate Attire:
- Wear only a towel or a swimsuit inside the sauna. Avoid wearing street clothes to maintain hygiene.

5. Keep Conversations Low:
- Maintain a quiet and peaceful atmosphere inside the sauna. If conversations are necessary, keep them at a low volume to avoid disturbing others.

6. Use a Towel as a Barrier:
- Sit or lie on your towel to create a barrier between your body and the sauna bench. This helps maintain cleanliness and prevents the spread of sweat.

7. Respect Personal Space:
- Be mindful of others' personal space. Leave enough room between yourself and others to allow for a comfortable and respectful experience.

8. Limit Session Duration:
- Respect recommended session durations and avoid staying in the sauna for extended periods. Long sessions can lead to dehydration.

9. Refrain from Bringing Food:
- Saunas are not the place for snacks. Refrain from bringing food inside to avoid mess and odors.

Exiting the Sauna:

10. Use Caution When Exiting:
- Be mindful of the heat when exiting the sauna. Take your time to acclimate to the temperature difference.

11. Cool Down Gradually:
- After leaving the sauna, cool down gradually by taking a lukewarm or cool shower. Avoid a sudden plunge into cold water.

General Etiquette:

12. Silence Your Phone:
- Keep your phone on silent mode or turn it off. Saunas are spaces for relaxation, and loud ringtones can be disruptive.

13. Avoid Strong Scents:
- Refrain from using strongly scented lotions, perfumes, or essential oils in the sauna, as they can affect others.

14. Respect Cultural Norms:
- In communal saunas, be aware of and respect any cultural norms or traditions that may differ from your own.

15. Practice Hygiene:
- If you have a contagious illness or infection, it's considerate to skip the sauna until you are no longer contagious.

16. Keep the Sauna Clean:
- Dispose of any used tissues or trash appropriately. Leave the sauna as clean as you found it.

17. Mind the Door:
- Close the sauna door gently to minimize disruptions. If there's a glass door, be aware of others in the sauna.

Mixed-Gender Saunas:

18. Respect Dress Codes:
- In mixed-gender saunas, respect any dress codes or guidelines provided. Be aware of and adhere to cultural expectations.

19. Use Separate Saunas:
- If separate saunas are available for men and women, use the designated areas to maintain privacy and comfort for all users.

Special Considerations:

20. Consult with Health Professionals:
- If you have health concerns or conditions, consult with a healthcare professional before using saunas.

21. Drink Plenty of Water:
- Stay hydrated by drinking water before and after sauna sessions. Avoid alcohol before using the sauna.

22. Know Your Limits:
- If you feel lightheaded or uncomfortable, exit the sauna and cool down. Listen to your body and know your limits.

11. Sauna Travel

Below, is a partial list of places around the world where you can experience authentic sauna culture. These places provide a snapshot of the diverse sauna cultures around the world, each with its own unique characteristics and traditions. Whether it's a historic bathhouse, a modern spa, or a traditional sauna in a natural setting, these locations offer authentic experiences for sauna enthusiasts. Keep in mind that the sauna culture can vary within countries and regions, so exploring different places will provide a rich understanding of the global sauna landscape.

Finland

1.
Löyly Sauna, Helsinki

Löyly Sauna in Helsinki encapsulates the essence of Finnish sauna culture, weaving together cultural, historical, and tourism elements. Its architectural prowess, commitment to tradition, and role as a wellness tourism hub make it not just a sauna but a living testament to Finland's cultural resilience and modern evolution. Whether one seeks the therapeutic warmth of traditional saunas or desires to bask in the architectural marvel of a contemporary urban retreat, Löyly offers an immersive experience that transcends time and tradition.

Cultural Significance:
Löyly Sauna stands as a contemporary ode to Finland's deep-rooted sauna culture. Positioned in Helsinki, a city intertwined with the sauna tradition, Löyly pays homage to both the historical significance and modern evolution of Finnish saunas. Saunas hold a sacred place in Finnish culture, serving as spaces for relaxation, socialization, and even decision-making. Löyly's presence in the heart of Helsinki reflects a commitment to preserving and advancing this cultural heritage.

Architectural Marvel:
The architectural design of Löyly is a marriage of tradition and innovation. Designed by Avanto Architects, the building's distinctive wooden façade mimics the texture of traditional Finnish wooden houses, creating a harmonious blend with its surroundings. The structure not only pays tribute to Finland's architectural heritage but also serves as a bold statement of modernity, symbolizing the nation's forward-looking approach to its cultural traditions.

Historical Roots:

In exploring the historical roots of Löyly Sauna, one uncovers the evolution of Finnish sauna practices. Historically, saunas were vital for physical and mental well-being, a place for communal gatherings, and a significant part of family life. Löyly's inclusion of both traditional Finnish saunas and a contemporary architectural setting mirrors the historical journey of saunas in Finland, evolving from modest structures to sophisticated urban retreats.

Tourist Attraction:

Löyly Sauna has become a must-visit destination for tourists seeking an authentic Finnish sauna experience. Its strategic location in the vibrant city of Helsinki ensures accessibility for visitors eager to immerse themselves in Finnish sauna culture. The blend of traditional and modern sauna offerings caters to a diverse audience, making Löyly an inclusive space where locals and tourists converge, fostering cultural exchange and shared sauna experiences.

Wellness Tourism Hub:

As wellness tourism gains prominence globally, Löyly Sauna positions itself as a wellness hub within Helsinki. Visitors seeking not only the therapeutic benefits of saunas but also a holistic urban retreat find solace in Löyly's serene atmosphere. The sauna's accessibility, coupled with its commitment to sustainability and architectural aesthetics, adds an extra layer to its appeal, making it a beacon for those in pursuit of well-being amidst the cultural and historical tapestry of Helsinki.

Environmental Consciousness:

Löyly Sauna goes beyond its role as a cultural and wellness destination; it embraces environmental consciousness. The use of sustainable building materials and eco-friendly practices aligns with Finland's commitment to environmental stewardship. This environmentally conscious approach adds a layer of cultural responsibility to Löyly's narrative, reflecting a modern ethos that respects tradition while embracing sustainability.

2.

Rajaportin Sauna, Tampere

Rajaportin Sauna in Tampere is more than a place to unwind; it is a time capsule that encapsulates the soul of Finnish sauna culture. Its historical roots, commitment to authenticity, and role as a community hub make it a treasure trove for those seeking not just a sauna experience but a profound journey into the heart of Finland's cultural and historical narrative.

Cultural Heritage:

Rajaportin Sauna in Tampere stands as a living testament to Finland's rich cultural heritage, specifically its enduring sauna tradition. Established in 1906, Rajaportin Sauna is recognized as the oldest public sauna in the country. Its cultural significance goes beyond its status as a place of relaxation; it is a cherished relic that embodies the communal spirit of Finnish sauna culture. Locals and visitors alike engage in a shared experience that transcends time, connecting with the roots of a tradition deeply ingrained in the Finnish way of life.

Historical Roots:
Dating back to the early 20th century, Rajaportin Sauna provides a glimpse into the historical evolution of saunas in Finland. At its inception, saunas were integral to daily life, serving as spaces for hygiene, socialization, and even as makeshift meeting rooms. Rajaportin Sauna preserves the architectural and cultural elements of that bygone era, allowing visitors to step back in time and experience the authenticity of Finnish sauna practices as they were over a century ago.

Authenticity of Experience:
What sets Rajaportin Sauna apart is its commitment to offering an authentic historical sauna experience. The building, with its traditional log structure, evokes a sense of nostalgia and transports visitors to an era when sauna bathing was a communal ritual deeply intertwined with daily life. The wood-burning stoves, rustic interiors, and the scent of burning wood contribute to an atmosphere that resonates with the soul of Finnish sauna traditions.

Tourist Attraction:
As a tourist attraction, Rajaportin Sauna draws visitors seeking a genuine immersion into Finnish culture and history. Tourists are not just patrons of a sauna; they become participants in a cultural narrative that predates modern Finland. The allure lies not only in the therapeutic benefits of sauna bathing but also in the unique opportunity to engage with a historical relic that continues to breathe life into age-old traditions.

Cultural Preservation:
Rajaportin Sauna serves as a custodian of cultural preservation, ensuring that the essence of Finnish sauna practices is not lost to the sands of time. Through meticulous maintenance of its historical architecture and adherence to traditional sauna customs, Rajaportin Sauna contributes to the ongoing dialogue about the importance of preserving cultural heritage in a rapidly changing world.

Community Hub:
Beyond its role as a tourist attraction, Rajaportin Sauna remains deeply embedded in the local community. It is a hub where Tampere residents continue to partake in a cultural legacy passed down through generations. The sauna's enduring popularity among locals speaks to its status not just as a historical relic

but as a vibrant, living entity that continues to foster community bonds and shared experiences.

3.

Saunasaari in the Helsinki Archipelago

Saunasaari in the Helsinki Archipelago is not just an island; it is a sanctuary where tradition meets tranquility. The traditional Finnish saunas, set against the backdrop of the archipelago's serene beauty, create a haven that transcends the ordinary. As visitors bask in the warmth of tradition amidst the natural symphony of Saunasaari, they embark on a journey that goes beyond relaxation—it is a cultural and natural immersion that lingers in the soul, inviting all to discover the harmonious dance between Finnish sauna practices and the enchanting allure of the Helsinki Archipelago.

Natural Oasis Near Helsinki:
Nestled in the embrace of the Helsinki Archipelago, Saunasaari emerges as an island sanctuary, inviting locals and visitors to escape the urban bustle and immerse themselves in the tranquil beauty of nature. Just a stone's throw away from the vibrant city, this island retreat offers a respite from the daily grind, beckoning all who seek solace in the soothing embrace of the natural world.

Traditional Finnish Sauna Haven:
Saunasaari is not merely an island; it is a haven of traditional Finnish saunas, seamlessly blending the timeless allure of sauna bathing with the raw beauty of its natural surroundings. The island's sauna offerings stay true to the authentic Finnish sauna experience, providing a sanctuary where the therapeutic warmth of tradition harmonizes with the peaceful ambiance of the archipelago.

Scenic Ambiance:
What sets Saunasaari apart is its scenic ambiance—an island canvas painted with the hues of pristine waters, lush greenery, and the whispers of the archipelago breeze. The saunas, strategically placed to offer panoramic views of the surrounding nature, create a sensory symphony where the therapeutic heat intertwines with the serenity of the archipelago landscape, providing a truly immersive experience.

Cultural Immersion:
Saunasaari invites visitors to not only indulge in sauna bathing but to immerse themselves in the cultural tapestry of Finnish island life. The island's ambiance, infused with the spirit of traditional saunas, serves as a cultural bridge, connecting those who venture here with the essence of Finnish sauna practices deeply ingrained in the nation's way of life.

Accessible Retreat:
The accessibility of Saunasaari adds to its allure. Situated near Helsinki, the island retreat becomes an accessible escape for both locals and tourists. Its proximity to the city allows individuals to seamlessly transition from the urban landscape to the serene island tranquility, creating a harmonious juxtaposition of experiences within a short journey from the heart of Helsinki.

Nature and Wellness Synergy:
Saunasaari embodies the synergy between nature and wellness. The island retreat doesn't just offer saunas; it provides an opportunity for individuals to reconnect with nature, fostering a holistic sense of well-being. Sauna sessions become a bridge to a mindful communion with the archipelago environment, where the therapeutic benefits of sauna bathing intertwine with the rejuvenating power of nature.

Sweden

Ribersborgs Kallbadhus in Malmo

Ribersborgs Kallbadhus in Malmo is not merely a bathhouse; it is a coastal sanctuary where history, tradition, and natural beauty converge. The blend of traditional saunas with Baltic Sea immersion creates an experience that transcends the ordinary, inviting all who enter to partake in the timeless dance between warmth and coolness, tradition and innovation, making it a haven of seaside serenity on the shores of Malmo.

Historical Charisma:
Perched on the shores of the Baltic Sea in Malmo, Ribersborgs Kallbadhus stands as a living testament to history, inviting visitors to step into a bygone era of seaside charm. The bathhouse, steeped in historical charisma, reflects the enduring allure of traditional Swedish bathing culture and stands as a timeless icon on the Malmo coastline.

Traditional Sauna Experience:
Ribersborgs Kallbadhus seamlessly blends tradition with tranquility, offering visitors an authentic Swedish sauna experience. The bathhouse preserves the essence of traditional saunas, where the wood-fired stoves infuse the air with the soothing scent of birch, creating an ambiance that harks back to the roots of Nordic bathing culture. Here, sauna bathing transcends the ordinary; it becomes a journey through time and tradition.

Baltic Sea Integration:
What sets Ribersborgs Kallbadhus apart is its unique integration of sauna bathing with the invigorating embrace of the Baltic Sea. Visitors have the opportunity to combine the therapeutic warmth of traditional saunas with refreshing dips in the cool Baltic waters. This seamless fusion of hot and cold, of relaxation and invigoration, creates a holistic and rejuvenating experience that defines the bathhouse's coastal charm.

Architectural Elegance:
The bathhouse's architectural elegance is a visual ode to both tradition and innovation. The building's design, reflecting a harmonious marriage of classic and contemporary elements, mirrors the dual nature of Ribersborgs Kallbadhus—a historic institution with a timeless allure that continues to evolve in sync with modern preferences. The panoramic views of the Baltic Sea from the bathhouse contribute to its aesthetic charm, creating an immersive experience for visitors.

Community Gathering Point:
Ribersborgs Kallbadhus is not just a bathhouse; it is a community gathering point where locals and visitors converge to partake in the communal ritual of seaside bathing. The bathhouse's social ambiance fosters a sense of community, where individuals from various walks of life come together to share the rejuvenating embrace of saunas and the Baltic Sea. This communal spirit adds an extra layer of warmth to the already inviting atmosphere.

Tourist Attraction:
As a tourist attraction, Ribersborgs Kallbadhus beckons travelers seeking an authentic Swedish experience. Its proximity to Malmo's city center and its historical significance make it a magnet for those eager to explore the cultural richness of the region. The bathhouse, with its blend of tradition, architectural splendor, and seaside setting, becomes a must-visit destination for tourists looking to immerse themselves in the unique coastal charm of Malmo.

Estonia

Saunamaa in Viljandi

Saunamaa in Viljandi is more than a collection of saunas; it is a cultural sanctuary where tradition meets diversity. The inclusion of traditional smoke saunas, the architectural harmony, and the commitment to wellness make Saunamaa a beacon for sauna enthusiasts and a vital contributor to the preservation of Estonia's sauna heritage. As visitors step into this Estonian sauna haven, they embark on a journey that transcends time, offering a glimpse into the soul of Estonia's sauna traditions.

Cultural Sauna Hub:
Nestled in the heart of Viljandi, Saunamaa emerges as a cultural sauna hub, inviting locals and visitors alike to experience the rich tapestry of Estonian sauna traditions. This sauna complex serves as a testament to Estonia's deep-rooted sauna culture, offering a multifaceted journey through the diverse world of sauna bathing, including the allure of traditional smoke saunas.

Variety of Sauna Experiences:
Saunamaa unfolds as a haven for sauna enthusiasts, boasting a diverse array of sauna experiences. From the comforting heat of traditional saunas to the distinct charm of smoke saunas, visitors can immerse themselves in a spectrum of sauna bathing styles. Each sauna, with its unique characteristics, becomes a portal to different facets of Estonian sauna heritage, ensuring a holistic and enriching experience for all who step through Saunamaa's doors.

Traditional Smoke Saunas:
The inclusion of traditional smoke saunas sets Saunamaa apart. These saunas, with their centuries-old roots, evoke a sense of nostalgia and authenticity. The gentle scent of wood smoke permeates the air, creating an atmosphere that harks back to Estonia's rural sauna traditions. Here, visitors can engage in a timeless ritual that connects them with the cultural and historical essence of Estonian sauna bathing.

Architectural Ambiance:
Saunamaa's architectural ambiance is a harmonious blend of modern comfort and traditional aesthetics. The sauna complex is designed to offer a cozy and inviting atmosphere, creating a space where visitors can unwind and reconnect with the timeless allure of sauna bathing. The architectural fusion captures the essence of Estonian sauna heritage while providing a contemporary setting for relaxation.

Wellness Oasis:
Saunamaa transcends the role of a traditional sauna complex; it becomes a wellness oasis in the heart of Viljandi. The variety of sauna experiences, coupled with the serene surroundings, offers visitors not just a physical retreat but a holistic journey toward well-being. The soothing heat, the scent of wood, and the tranquil environment contribute to a sensory symphony that rejuvenates both body and spirit.

Cultural Preservation:
As a guardian of Estonian sauna traditions, Saunamaa plays a crucial role in cultural preservation. By offering a diverse range of saunas, including traditional smoke saunas, the complex becomes a living museum of Estonia's sauna heritage. Visitors engage in more than a leisurely activity; they become participants in the preservation of a cultural legacy that spans generations.

Local and Tourist Appeal:
Saunamaa is not just a local gem; it also beckons to tourists seeking an authentic Estonian experience. Its strategic location in Viljandi, a city known for its historical charm, positions Saunamaa as a cultural landmark where locals and tourists converge to partake in the shared ritual of sauna bathing. The complex's cultural and architectural significance adds an extra layer of appeal for those eager to explore Estonia's sauna traditions.

Russia

Sanduny Banya in Moscow

Sanduny Banya in Moscow is a time capsule of Russian sauna culture, where history, tradition, and opulence converge. As patrons step through its ornate doors, they embark on a journey that transcends centuries, immersing themselves in the enduring legacy of Moscow's most famous bathhouse. Sanduny stands as a living testament to the cultural richness of Russian sauna traditions and a symbol of Moscow's unwavering connection to its historical roots

Timeless Elegance:
Nestled in the heart of Moscow, Sanduny Banya stands as a paragon of historical grandeur, inviting patrons to step into a bygone era of Russian bathing traditions. Dating back to the 19th century, this iconic bathhouse is not merely a place of relaxation; it is a living testament to Moscow's rich cultural heritage, offering a timeless escape from the hustle and bustle of the modern world.

Architectural Splendor:
The architectural splendor of Sanduny Banya is a symphony of opulence and tradition. The building's design reflects the elegance of the 19th century, adorned with intricate details that transport visitors to a different epoch. The ornate interiors, grand halls, and meticulously preserved elements create an ambiance that is both regal and inviting, contributing to the overall allure of Sanduny Banya as a cultural treasure.

Oldest Bathhouse in Moscow:
As one of the oldest bathhouses in Moscow, Sanduny Banya holds a distinguished status in the city's historical landscape. Its longevity is a testament to the enduring appeal of the traditional Russian banya experience. Generation after generation, patrons have sought refuge in the soothing heat of Sanduny's saunas, making it a cultural institution deeply ingrained in the fabric of Moscow's communal life.

Traditional Russian Banya Experience:
Sanduny Banya offers a quintessential Russian *banya* experience that transcends time. The wood-burning stoves, the invigorating steam, and the distinct rituals echo the age-old traditions of Russian sauna culture. Here, visitors partake in more than a leisurely activity; they immerse themselves in a cultural practice that has withstood the test of time, fostering a sense of connection to Russia's historical roots.

Cultural Icon and Landmark:
Sanduny Banya is not just a bathhouse; it is a cultural icon and a landmark that defines Moscow's architectural and historical landscape. Locals and tourists alike are drawn to its allure, eager to experience the rituals and ambiance that have been cherished for over a century. The bathhouse's role as a cultural touchstone makes it an essential stop for those seeking to unravel the layers of Moscow's rich history.

Luxurious Retreat:
While rooted in tradition, Sanduny Banya also exudes an air of luxury. The bathhouse offers patrons an indulgent retreat where they can revel in the opulence of historic surroundings. From ornate relaxation rooms to elaborate mosaic-covered chambers, Sanduny provides a luxurious backdrop for the traditional banya experience, elevating it to a level of refinement that is both decadent and culturally significant.

Wellness and Social Hub:
Beyond its historical and architectural significance, Sanduny Banya serves as a wellness and social hub in Moscow. Patrons not only come for the therapeutic benefits of sauna bathing but also for the communal spirit that permeates the bathhouse. The shared experience of relaxation, conversation, and rejuvenation fosters a sense of community, making Sanduny not just a place to unwind but a communal sanctuary.

Japan

Dogo Onsen in Matsuyama

Dogo Onsen in Matsuyama is a living chapter in Japan's bathing legacy. Its cultural significance, architectural splendor, and role as a haven of wellness make it not just a hot spring but a timeless symbol of Japan's commitment to preserving its cultural heritage. As patrons step into Dogo Onsen, they embark on a journey through time, where the soothing waters carry the whispers of centuries-old traditions and the art of communal bathing is celebrated with grace and reverence.

Historical Oasis:
Nestled in Matsuyama, Dogo Onsen is a revered sanctuary and a testament to Japan's enduring bathing culture. As one of the oldest hot springs in the country, it unveils a historical oasis where visitors are invited to immerse themselves in the gentle embrace of thermal waters, creating an experience that transcends mere bathing—it becomes a journey into the heart of Japanese tradition.

Cultural Legacy:
Dogo Onsen is more than a hot spring; it is a living embodiment of Japan's bathing legacy. Steeped in history, this *onsen* has been a cultural cornerstone for centuries, witnessing the ebb and flow of time while maintaining its role as a custodian of Japanese bathing traditions. The architectural elegance of Dogo Onsen reflects the nation's commitment to preserving its cultural heritage, providing visitors with a rare glimpse into the refined past of Japanese communal bathing.

Architectural Marvel:
The architectural marvel of Dogo Onsen is a fusion of elegance and tradition. The iconic three-story wooden structure, known as the main building, stands as a symbol of Japanese *onsen* culture. With its intricate lattice windows and nostalgic charm, the building transports visitors to a time when communal bathing was not just a physical activity but a ritual deeply intertwined with societal and cultural nuances.

Unique Bathing Culture:
Dogo Onsen offers a unique bathing culture that goes beyond the ordinary. The *onsen* experience here is not solely about the thermal waters; it is a harmonious blend of ambiance, ritual, and tradition. The distinct charm lies in the meticulous rituals observed, from the symbolic purification at the entrance to the communal enjoyment of the thermal waters. Every step in Dogo Onsen unfolds as a cultural dance, connecting patrons to the refined art of Japanese bathing.

Literary and Cinematic Inspiration:
Dogo Onsen's allure extends beyond its physical presence; it has inspired literary works and cinematic masterpieces. The famed Japanese writer Natsume Soseki drew inspiration from Dogo Onsen in his novel "Botchan," elevating the *onsen* to a literary icon. Furthermore, the *onsen's* appearance in Studio Ghibli's animated film "Spirited Away" solidified its status as a cultural touchstone, captivating audiences worldwide and adding an extra layer of enchantment to its legacy.

Healing Waters and Wellness:
The thermal waters of Dogo *Onsen* are believed to possess healing properties, contributing to the *onsen's* reputation as a wellness destination. Visitors not only

indulge in the sensory delights of the bath but also seek the therapeutic benefits attributed to the mineral-rich waters. The *onsen* experience becomes a holistic journey, promoting physical and mental well-being amidst the cultural tapestry of Matsuyama.

Tourist and Local Magnet:
Dogo Onsen's magnetic pull extends to both tourists and locals. While it captivates international visitors eager to partake in a quintessential Japanese *onsen* experience, it remains an integral part of local life. The *onsen* serves as a communal hub where residents gather to unwind, fostering a sense of community and continuity in Matsuyama's cultural narrative.

United States

Glen Ivy Hot Springs

Glen Ivy Hot Springs in California is more than a spa—it is a holistic wellness destination where nature, hot springs, saunas, and a myriad of activities converge. The spa's commitment to providing a diverse and customizable wellness experience makes it a haven for those seeking not just relaxation but a comprehensive journey toward physical and mental well-being. As patrons immerse themselves in the warm waters and embrace the wellness offerings, Glen Ivy becomes a retreat where the spirit of California's wellness culture comes to life.

Natural Retreat:
Nestled in the heart of California, Glen Ivy Hot Springs emerges as an oasis of tranquility, drawing patrons into the embrace of natural hot springs and a holistic spa experience. Surrounded by scenic landscapes, this destination invites visitors to unwind and rejuvenate in a setting that harmonizes with the spirit of wellness.

Hot Springs Haven:
Glen Ivy's claim to fame lies in its natural hot springs, which have been a source of relaxation and healing for centuries. The geothermally heated waters provide a therapeutic haven, offering patrons a unique opportunity to soak in the warmth and mineral-rich embrace of the springs. This natural feature becomes the cornerstone of the spa experience, providing a rejuvenating escape from the demands of modern life.

Sauna Serenity:
Complementing the hot springs, Glen Ivy features saunas that add a layer of serenity to the spa experience. The saunas, with their varying temperatures and styles, cater to different preferences, allowing visitors to tailor their wellness journey.

From traditional dry saunas to steam rooms, each enclave becomes a retreat for relaxation and cleansing, contributing to the overall sense of well-being.

Wellness Activities Galore:
Glen Ivy Hot Springs goes beyond the conventional spa experience by offering a plethora of wellness activities. Visitors can engage in yoga sessions, fitness classes, and mindfulness activities, creating a comprehensive approach to well-being. The spa's commitment to holistic health is evident in the diverse range of activities, ensuring that patrons can customize their experience to align with their personal wellness goals.

Scenic Surroundings:
The spa's location in California's picturesque landscape adds an extra layer of enchantment to the Glen Ivy experience. Surrounded by lush greenery and complemented by open-air spaces, the spa becomes a retreat where patrons not only indulge in wellness activities but also connect with nature. The scenic surroundings contribute to a sense of serenity and mindfulness, elevating the overall spa journey.

Variety of Experiences:
Glen Ivy Hot Springs caters to a diverse audience by offering a variety of experiences. Whether visitors seek quiet relaxation, active pursuits, or social interactions, the spa provides spaces and activities that accommodate different preferences. The versatility of Glen Ivy's offerings ensures that each visitor can craft a spa experience that aligns with their unique wellness needs.

Community Wellness Hub:
Beyond being a spa, Glen Ivy Hot Springs serves as a community wellness hub. Locals and tourists converge to partake in the shared pursuit of well-being, fostering a sense of community. The spa becomes a space where individuals connect over a common commitment to health, creating a vibrant atmosphere that transcends the boundaries of traditional spa experiences.

Canada

Scandinave Spa, Whistler

Scandinave Spa in Whistler is more than a destination—it is a Nordic-inspired sanctuary where the spirit of Scandinavian wellness traditions merges with the awe-inspiring beauty of the Canadian Rockies. Patrons embark on a holistic journey of hydrotherapy, sauna rituals, and silent serenity, creating an experience that transcends the ordinary spa visit. As visitors surrender to the rhythms of nature and the therapeutic embrace of the spa, Scandinave Spa becomes a haven where the rejuvenating essence of Nordic traditions meets the majestic allure of Whistler's mountainous landscapes.

Nordic Oasis in Nature:
Nestled amidst the breathtaking scenery of the Canadian Rockies, the Scandinave Spa in Whistler emerges as a Nordic-inspired oasis of tranquility. Drawing inspiration from Scandinavian spa traditions, this wellness retreat offers patrons a unique opportunity to harmonize with nature while indulging in a rejuvenating hydrotherapy experience.

Traditional Scandinavian Hydrotherapy:
At the heart of the Scandinave Spa experience lies the essence of traditional Scandinavian hydrotherapy. The spa takes patrons on a sensory journey that alternates between hot and cold elements—a practice deeply rooted in Nordic wellness traditions. From saunas that embrace the warmth of wood-fired stoves to invigorating cold plunges, visitors engage in a ritual that promotes relaxation, rejuvenation, and the beneficial effects of hydrotherapy.

Sauna Sanctuary:
The Scandinave Spa in Whistler is a sanctuary of saunas, each contributing to the overall warmth and serenity of the experience. From traditional dry saunas to eucalyptus-infused steam rooms, patrons have the opportunity to explore various sauna styles, each with its unique therapeutic benefits. The sauna circuit becomes a ritual of purification, promoting detoxification and a profound sense of calm.

Cold Plunge Revitalization:
As an integral part of the hydrotherapy experience, Scandinave Spa introduces patrons to the invigorating practice of cold plunges. The contrast between the heated saunas and the refreshing cold plunges enhances circulation, reduces muscle inflammation, and adds an exhilarating dimension to the spa journey. This juxtaposition of temperatures becomes a key element in the Nordic-inspired wellness philosophy.

Nature-Infused Design:
The design of Scandinave Spa in Whistler is a reflection of its commitment to nature-infused tranquility. Surrounded by evergreen forests and mountain vistas, the spa's architecture seamlessly blends with its natural surroundings. Outdoor installations, including thermal waterfalls and relaxation areas, allow patrons to immerse themselves in the pristine beauty of the Canadian Rockies while embracing the Nordic spa experience.

Silent Serenity:
A unique aspect of the Scandinave Spa experience is the dedication to maintaining a silent environment. Visitors are encouraged to embrace the serene atmosphere by minimizing conversation, fostering a space for introspection and mindfulness. The silent serenity adds an extra layer of tranquility to the spa journey, allowing patrons to connect with their inner selves amidst the soothing embrace of nature.

Year-Round Wellness Retreat:
Scandinave Spa in Whistler is not bound by seasonal limitations. Operating year-round, the spa offers a different yet equally enchanting experience in every season. From the snow-covered landscapes of winter to the vibrant colors of summer, patrons can immerse themselves in the Nordic-inspired wellness retreat regardless of the time of year, creating a dynamic and ever-evolving spa escape.

Germany

Liquidrom, Berlin

Liquidrom in Berlin is not merely a spa; it is a contemporary wellness destination that marries architectural innovation with multisensory indulgence. The futuristic floating pool, sauna spectacle, and commitment to urban retreat redefine the spa experience. As patrons navigate the modern aesthetics and immerse themselves in the multisensory journey, Liquidrom becomes a haven where the future of wellness unfolds in the heart of Berlin's dynamic urban landscape.

Urban Wellness Oasis:
Tucked away in the vibrant cityscape of Berlin, Liquidrom emerges as a modern spa haven, inviting patrons to escape the hustle and bustle of urban life and indulge in a unique wellness experience. This oasis of tranquility seamlessly blends contemporary design with futuristic elements, creating an urban retreat that transcends the ordinary.

Architectural Innovation:
At the core of Liquidrom's allure is its architectural innovation. The spa's design embraces modernity, featuring sleek lines, minimalist aesthetics, and a harmonious integration of glass and steel. This architectural finesse creates an ambiance that reflects Berlin's avant-garde spirit, setting the stage for a spa experience that is as visually captivating as it is restorative.

Futuristic Floating Pool:
The centerpiece of Liquidrom's uniqueness is its futuristic floating pool—a visual

and sensory masterpiece. Patrons are invited to submerge themselves in the ethereal tranquility of the pool, where ambient music and underwater sounds add an immersive dimension to the experience. The futuristic design of the pool becomes a symbol of Liquidrom's commitment to pushing the boundaries of traditional spa offerings.

Sauna Spectacle:
Liquidrom redefines the sauna experience, introducing patrons to a spectacle of heat and relaxation. The spa features a variety of saunas, each with its unique theme and ambiance. From traditional Finnish saunas to herbal steam rooms, visitors can embark on a sauna circuit that caters to different preferences. The sauna journey becomes a ritual of rejuvenation, promoting detoxification and a profound sense of well-being.

Multisensory Wellness:
Liquidrom's commitment to multisensory wellness is evident in every facet of the spa experience. The integration of visual arts, ambient music, and unique lighting designs transforms the space into a multisensory playground. Patrons are not just bathers; they become participants in an immersive journey that engages all the senses, fostering a deeper connection between mind, body, and environment.

Underwater Soundscapes:
One of the standout features of Liquidrom is its emphasis on underwater soundscapes. As patrons float in the futuristic pool or relax in the saunas, they are enveloped in a symphony of soothing sounds. This underwater auditory experience elevates the spa journey, creating a sense of serenity that is both unique and indulgent.

Wellness Events and Performances:
Liquidrom transcends the traditional spa model by hosting wellness events and performances. From live music to ambient performances, the spa becomes a venue for cultural and wellness convergence. Patrons can immerse themselves in a holistic experience that goes beyond the typical spa visit, adding an element of cultural enrichment to their wellness journey.

Cityscape Retreat:
Liquidrom's strategic location within Berlin transforms it into a cityscape retreat. Surrounded by the urban energy of the city, the spa becomes a refuge where patrons can recalibrate their senses and find respite. The juxtaposition of city life and spa serenity creates a unique dynamic, offering visitors a moment of escape without leaving the heart of Berlin.

Norway

The Well, Oslo

The Well in Oslo is more than a spa; it is a Nordic sanctuary where patrons can e scape the demands of daily life and immerse themselves in the rich tapestry of Scandinavian wellness traditions. From the sauna rituals that pay homage to Nordic heritage to the architectural elegance that mirrors the surrounding nature, The Well becomes a retreat where the essence of Nordic tranquility unfolds. As visitors surrender to the sauna heat, embrace the natural surroundings, and indulge in holistic well-being, The Well stands as a testament to Norway's commitment to providing a wellness sanctuary that resonates with the soul.

Nestled in Nature:
Situated near Oslo, The Well emerges as a serene spa and wellness center, nestled amidst the natural beauty of Norway. The spa's strategic location integrates seamlessly with the surrounding landscape, inviting patrons to embark on a wellness journey that harmonizes with the tranquility of Nordic nature.

Nordic Sauna Traditions:
At the heart of The Well's allure is its homage to Nordic bathing traditions. The spa features a range of saunas, each inspired by the rich heritage of Scandinavian wellness rituals. From traditional Finnish saunas to innovative variations, visitors are enveloped in the authentic warmth and therapeutic benefits that define Nordic sauna culture.

Architectural Elegance:
The architectural design of The Well is a testament to Nordic elegance. Surrounded by lush greenery and adorned with contemporary Scandinavian aesthetics, the spa seamlessly blends modern comfort with traditional charm. The architecture becomes an extension of the spa's commitment to providing a holistic experience that appeals to both the senses and the soul.

Sauna Sanctuary:
The Well's sauna sanctuary is a haven for those seeking relaxation and rejuvenation. Patrons can explore a variety of saunas, each offering a distinctive atmosphere and experience. Whether it's the dry heat of a traditional sauna or the aromatic infusion of a steam room, visitors can tailor their sauna journey to suit their preferences, creating a personalized retreat within the spa.

Nature-Inspired Retreat Areas:
Complementing the sauna experience, The Well provides nature-inspired retreat areas. Outdoor spaces, relaxation zones, and terraces allow patrons to connect

with nature while enjoying the spa's amenities. The serene environment enhances the overall wellness journey, offering moments of quiet contemplation and connection with the Nordic surroundings.

Thermal Pools and Water Rituals:
The Well's dedication to thermal pools and water rituals transforms the spa experience into a fluid and immersive journey. From the rejuvenating warmth of thermal baths to the invigorating plunge into refreshing pools, each element is a carefully orchestrated note in the symphony of Nordic wellness. As visitors submerge themselves in this aquatic sanctuary, they emerge not only refreshed but also rejuvenated, having embraced the therapeutic embrace of water in a way that is uniquely synonymous with The Well's commitment to holistic wellness.

Hydrotherapy Rituals:
The art of hydrotherapy takes center stage at The Well, where patrons are invited to indulge in a variety of water-based rituals. From gentle cascading waterfalls that massage and invigorate to strategically placed jets that target specific muscle groups, each hydrotherapy feature is a carefully crafted element in the spa's dedication to holistic well-being. Hydrotherapy becomes a choreographed dance of water, promoting relaxation, improving flexibility, and contributing to the overall sense of rejuvenation.

Seasonal Wellness:
The Well adapts to the changing seasons, offering a different yet equally enchanting experience throughout the year. From the crisp freshness of winter to the vibrant colors of summer, patrons can immerse themselves in a spa retreat that aligns with the distinctive beauty of each season, creating a dynamic and ever-evolving wellness experience.

Culinary Delights:
Beyond the wellness offerings, The Well extends its commitment to holistic well-being with culinary delights. The spa's restaurant curates a menu that emphasizes fresh, locally sourced ingredients, providing visitors with a gastronomic journey that complements their overall wellness experience. The integration of nourishing food enhances the spa's dedication to holistic health.

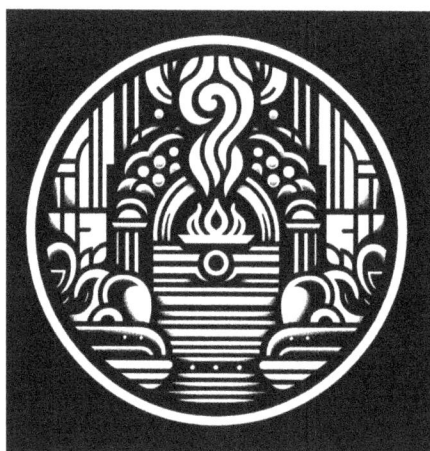

1. The Universal Appeal of Steam: A Cross-Cultural Exploration

Steam, with its ethereal tendrils rising gracefully, has captivated human senses for millennia. The universal appeal of steam transcends cultural boundaries, weaving itself into the fabric of diverse societies worldwide. Beyond its physical properties, steam holds symbolic, spiritual, and therapeutic significance, creating a shared experience that resonates across the epochs.

Steam's Elemental Allure:
At its essence, steam is an elemental force – a dance between water and heat. This fundamental interplay, observable in the billowing geysers of Yellowstone, the misty hot springs of Iceland, and the cozy hearths of ancient homes, is inherently linked to the human experience. The hiss of steam escaping from a pot, the comforting warmth of a sauna, or the rhythmic rise and fall of steam in a traditional tea ceremony – these manifestations of steam speak to our primal connection with the elements.

Practical and Mystical Utility in Ancient Times:
In ancient Mesopotamia, where civilizations burgeoned along the Tigris and Euphrates, the *Hammams* of Babylon served not only as bathhouses but as centers of communal life. The rising steam symbolized cleansing – a physical and spiritual purging that found echoes in rituals and religious practices. Similarly, in the heart of ancient Egypt, the use of steam in bathhouses became an integral part of healing rituals, mirroring the dualistic nature of the Nile as a life-giving force and a symbol of transformation.

The Greco-Roman world, known for its philosophical depth and cultural richness, embraced steam in bathhouses like the Roman *thermae*. Steam, in this context, was not merely a means of physical cleansing but a conduit for intellectual exchange. The Far East, with its distinct cultural tapestry, infused steam into traditional practices such as the Japanese *Onsen* and Chinese steam baths. Here, steam was both a medium of physical rejuvenation and a channel for spiritual connection with nature.

Indigenous Wisdom and Shared Symbolism:
Indigenous cultures, scattered across continents, embraced steam in diverse ways. Native American sweat lodges were spaces where steam became a tool for communal bonding and spiritual introspection. In Australia, Indigenous communities engaged in steam rituals, weaving Dreamtime stories into the fabric of their practices. The cross-cultural influences facilitated by ancient trade routes led to shared symbolism – the universal acknowledgment of steam as a symbol of transformation, renewal, and communal gathering.

The Common Thread of Purification:
One common thread that unites these diverse manifestations is the concept of purification. The rising steam, carrying away impurities, symbolizes not just the cleansing of the physical body but also the purification of the soul. This shared symbolism underscores the universal human yearning for renewal and transformation – a timeless pursuit embedded in the rising vapors that blur the boundaries between the material and the metaphysical.

From Ancient Practices to Modern Wellness:
As civilizations evolved, so did the ways in which steam was incorporated into daily life. The public bathhouses of the 18th century in Europe and the hammams of the Ottoman Empire continued the legacy of communal steam experiences. Steam became intertwined with hygiene, socialization, and even political discourse. The Industrial Revolution brought steam to the forefront of technological advancement, a symbol of progress and power.

In the 20th century, steam found its place in modern medicine, with steam therapy becoming a recognized form of treatment. The sauna, originating from ancient practices, became a staple in wellness centers worldwide. Today, the universal appeal of steam persists in contemporary spa culture, where steam rooms provide sanctuary for relaxation and rejuvenation.

Symbolic Resonance in Modern Times:
Beyond its practical applications, the symbolic resonance of steam endures. The rising steam in a modern urban coffee shop, the steam that envelops a yoga studio during a heated practice, or the steam rising from a pot of herbal tea – these instances echo the ancient symbolism of renewal and transformation. Steam, in its myriad forms, continues to be a bridge between the physical and the metaphysical, a reminder of our elemental connection to the world and each other.

2. Steam History

Ancient Mesopotamia: *Hammams* of Babylon

In the cradle of civilization, where the Tigris and Euphrates rivers wove the fertile plains of Mesopotamia, a distinct tradition of communal bathing emerged. The *Hammams* of Babylon, enigmatic and steeped in history, stand as testament to the sophistication of ancient Mesopotamian societies.

Architectural Marvels:

The *Hammams* of Babylon were architectural marvels, intricately designed structures that transcended the utilitarian aspect of bathing. These communal bathhouses were not merely places to cleanse the body; they were centers of social, cultural, and spiritual life. The architectural grandeur reflected the advanced engineering capabilities of Mesopotamian civilizations, showcasing their ability to manipulate water for both practical and symbolic purposes.

Ritualistic Ceremonies:

Within the walls of the *Hammams,* ritualistic ceremonies unfolded, weaving a tapestry of communal practices. The process of bathing was elevated beyond a mundane act; it became a sacred ritual. The *Hammams* were spaces where the physical and the metaphysical converged, where the act of cleansing the body was entwined with spiritual significance.

Water as a Symbol of Purification:

Water, in Mesopotamian culture, held profound symbolism. The *Hammams* were adorned with intricate carvings and murals depicting water as a purifying force. The symbolic cleansing associated with water extended beyond the physical realm, echoing the Mesopotamian belief in the transformative power of ritualistic bathing.

Religious Significance:

The *Hammams* of Babylon were not just communal spaces but sacred precincts intertwined with religious practices. Rituals performed within these bathhouses were often accompanied by invocations to deities associated with water and purification. The act of cleansing oneself in the *Hammams* became a form of spiritual devotion, a way to seek favor from divine entities and ensure spiritual well-being.

Social Cohesion and Intellectual Exchange:

Beyond their religious and spiritual functions, the *Hammams* served as hubs for social cohesion and intellectual exchange. In the warm embrace of steam, people engaged in conversations, forging bonds and sharing ideas. The *Hammams* became microcosms of Mesopotamian society, where the boundaries between social, spiritual, and intellectual realms blurred, creating a holistic environment for communal well-being.

Legacy and Influence:

The legacy of the *Hammams* of Babylon extended far beyond the confines of Mesopotamia. As trade routes flourished, so did the influence of these bathhouses on neighboring cultures. The *Hammams* became symbols of Mesopotamian sophistication and contributed to the broader narrative of communal bathing practices in the ancient world.

The *Hammams* of Babylon, with their ritualistic ceremonies and religious significance, offer a glimpse into the multi-faceted nature of ancient Mesopotamian societies. These bathhouses were more than architectural wonders; they were sacred spaces where the physical, spiritual, and social dimensions of life converged. The legacy of the *Hammams* resonates through time, reminding us of the profound connection between communal bathing, spirituality, and the intricate tapestry of ancient civilizations.

Ancient Egypt: The Mystique of Egyptian Bathhouses

In the sun-kissed land of the Nile, where monumental pyramids and majestic temples adorned the landscape, the ancient Egyptians crafted a civilization steeped in mysticism and sophistication. Within this rich tapestry of history, Egyptian bathhouses emerged as centers of communal life, imbued with an aura of mystique that transcended the realms of mere physical cleansing.

Architectural Grandeur:
Egyptian bathhouses were not ordinary structures; they were architectural marvels designed with precision and adorned with intricate carvings. These bathhouses, often located near temples and palaces, mirrored the grandeur of Egyptian civilization. The walls were adorned with hieroglyphs and depictions of deities, emphasizing the sacred nature of the bathing rituals.

Mystical Symbolism:
The mystique of Egyptian bathhouses lay in the mystical symbolism associated with water. In Egyptian cosmology, water was a primordial force, a symbol of creation and rejuvenation. The act of bathing took on a sacred dimension, aligning with the cosmic order and the cycles of life and death. The very process of
entering the bathhouse became a symbolic journey of purification and renewal.

Purification Rituals:
Egyptian bathhouses were not merely places for physical cleansing; they were spaces for elaborate purification rituals. The use of steam was an integral part of these rituals, symbolizing the transformative power of water. The rising steam, enveloping bathers in a warm embrace, was believed to cleanse not just the body but also the spirit, paving the way for spiritual ascent.

Role of Steam in Healing Practices:
Steam played a pivotal role in Egyptian healing practices, seamlessly integrated

into the broader tapestry of holistic well-being. The therapeutic properties of steam were harnessed for a myriad of health benefits. The warmth of the steam was believed to soothe muscles, alleviate respiratory ailments, and promote overall vitality. Egyptian healers recognized the symbiotic relationship between physical and spiritual health, and steam became a conduit for achieving equilibrium in both realms.

Connection to Deities:
The mystical ambiance of Egyptian bathhouses extended to their connection with deities. Bathing rituals were often accompanied by invocations to water deities such as Hapi, the god of the Nile, or more precisely, the inundation event of the Nile, and Isis, associated with healing and magic. The steam-filled chambers became spaces where the divine and the mortal converged, where individuals sought not only physical rejuvenation but also divine blessings.

Social and Intellectual Exchange:
Egyptian bathhouses were vibrant hubs for social interaction and intellectual exchange. As bathers luxuriated in the soothing warmth of the steam, conversations flowed, ideas were exchanged, and bonds were forged. The bathhouses became microcosms of Egyptian society, reflecting the interconnectedness of physical well-being, spirituality, and communal life.

Enduring Legacy:
The mystique of Egyptian bathhouses left an enduring legacy that resonates through the annals of history. As trade routes connected civilizations, the influence of Egyptian bathing practices spread far beyond the banks of the Nile. The symbolism, rituals, and healing traditions associated with Egyptian bathhouses continue to inspire contemporary wellness practices.

The mystique of Egyptian bathhouses, with their elaborate rituals and the integral role of steam in healing practices, unveils a captivating chapter in the narrative of ancient Egyptian civilization. Beyond the architectural grandeur, these bathhouses were portals to a world where the physical, spiritual, and communal dimensions of life converged in a harmonious dance, leaving an indelible mark on the cultural tapestry of antiquity.

Greco-Roman Civilization: Bathhouses in Ancient Greece

In the heart of Ancient Greece, where philosophy, art, and civic life flourished, bathhouses held a central place in daily routines and cultural practices. These communal spaces were not merely for physical cleansing but were arenas for social interaction, philosophical discourse, and an exploration of the human experience.

Philosophical Foundations:

Bathhouses in Ancient Greece were more than utilitarian structures; they were embodiments of philosophical ideals. The Greeks, recognizing the harmony between physical and intellectual well-being, viewed bathing as a holistic practice. Bathhouses were places where the body and mind converged, creating an environment conducive to both relaxation and intellectual exchange.

Athletic and Cultural Significance:

Bathhouses in Ancient Greece were not solely places of leisure; they were extensions of the gymnasiums, spaces dedicated to physical fitness and intellectual pursuits. Athletes engaged in oil massages and scraped off dirt and sweat in the baths, fostering a culture that celebrated the athletic body. Moreover, bathhouses became venues for cultural discussions, where poets, philosophers, and citizens gathered to share ideas.

Water as a Symbol of Purity:

In Ancient Greece, water held profound symbolic significance. The act of bathing represented not only physical purification but also a spiritual cleansing. The communal pools and steam rooms were places where individuals sought to cleanse not just their bodies but also their souls, fostering a connection between the corporeal and the metaphysical.

Hygienic Practices:

While the Greeks embraced the philosophical and symbolic aspects of bathing, there was a pragmatic side to it as well. Hygiene and cleanliness were paramount, especially in a society that valued physical prowess and aesthetic ideals. Bathing became a ritualized practice, with elaborate processes involving oils, scrubs, and massages.

Roman *Thermae* and Public Bathing Culture

With the rise of the Roman Empire, the bathing culture of Ancient Greece underwent a grand transformation, evolving into the iconic Roman *thermae* – colossal structures that reflected the engineering prowess and opulence of the Roman civilization.

Architectural Extravagance:

Roman *thermae* were architectural marvels, boasting expansive halls, intricate mosaics, and intricate frescoes. These structures were not merely places to cleanse the body; they were sprawling complexes that included libraries, gardens, and exercise areas. The grandeur of the Roman *thermae* was a testament to the empire's wealth and commitment to public welfare.

Social Hubs:
Roman *thermae* were integral to Roman social life. They served as communal spaces where individuals from all walks of life converged. The egalitarian nature of Roman bathing culture allowed citizens, regardless of social status, to access the *thermae*, fostering a sense of community and shared experience.

Cultural and Intellectual Nexus:
Similar to their Greek predecessors, the Romans viewed the baths as spaces for more than just physical cleansing. The *thermae* became hubs for cultural and intellectual exchange. Romans engaged in discussions, debates, and even conducted business within the confines of these grand bathing establishments. The baths were spaces where the social fabric of Roman society was woven.

Technological Ingenuity:
The Roman *thermae* were not only symbols of luxury but also feats of engineering. Elaborate systems of aqueducts and heating mechanisms ensured a constant supply of hot water for the baths. The *hypocaust*, an underfloor heating system, transformed the bathing experience, allowing Romans to indulge in warm baths even during colder seasons.

Public Health and Ritualized Practices:
Roman bathing culture was deeply ingrained in notions of public health. The regular use of the *thermae* was seen as a preventive measure against illness, and the act of bathing became a ritualized practice. Romans engaged in a sequence of activities, including the *caldarium* (hot bath), *tepidarium* (warm bath), and *frigidarium* (cold plunge), adhering to a prescribed order for maximum health benefits.

Enduring Legacy:
The Greco-Roman bathing culture, with its philosophical foundations and architectural marvels, left an enduring legacy that echoes through time. The communal and intellectual aspects of bathing practiced in these ancient civilizations continue to influence contemporary notions of wellness and community.

The bathhouses of Ancient Greece and the Roman *thermae* were not merely spaces for physical cleansing; they were cultural phenomena that encapsulated the ideals, aspirations, and societal structures of their respective civilizations. From philosophical musings in the Greek baths to the opulent grandeur of Roman *thermae*, these communal spaces were integral to the fabric of Greco-Roman society, leaving an indelible mark on the history of communal bathing.

Far East: Traditional Chinese Steam Baths

In the Far East, where ancient traditions and holistic approaches to well-being thrived, the practice of bathing extended beyond physical cleansing to encompass spiritual rejuvenation. Traditional Chinese steam baths, deeply rooted in ancient Chinese culture, were spaces where the interplay of heat and steam was harnessed not only for bodily health but also for spiritual balance.

Philosophical Foundations:
Traditional Chinese steam baths were imbued with the principles of Traditional Chinese Medicine (TCM). The philosophy of achieving harmony between the body's vital forces, known as *Qi*, and the opposing forces of Yin and Yang, shaped the approach to bathing. The steam, with its warming properties, was seen as a means of balancing these fundamental energies within the body.

Meridian Therapy and Acupressure:
The Chinese steam bath experience was often enriched by practices such as meridian therapy and acupressure. Steam was believed to open the body's meridians, allowing the flow of Qi to be unblocked. Concurrently, acupressure points were stimulated, aligning with TCM principles to promote overall well-being.

Herbal Infusions and Aromatherapy:
Herbal infusions and aromatherapy played a significant role in Chinese steam baths. Steam chambers were often infused with medicinal herbs like ginseng, eucalyptus, and ginger, enhancing the therapeutic benefits of the experience. The aromatic steam not only invigorated the senses but also contributed to the holistic healing properties of the bath.

Spiritual and Therapeutic Dimensions:
Beyond its physical benefits, the Chinese steam bath held spiritual dimensions. The act of bathing was considered a ritual, a time for introspection and reconnection with one's inner self. The rising steam became a metaphor for the ascent of one's spirit, creating a serene space for mental and emotional rejuvenation.

Japanese Onsen and Spiritual Cleansing

In Japan, a country shaped by its unique blend of Shinto and Buddhist traditions, the *onsen*, or hot springs, hold a revered place in cultural practices. Far more than places for mere physical cleansing, *onsen* are sacred sites where the interplay of natural hot water and pristine surroundings is believed to cleanse both body and soul.

Sacred Geothermal Springs:
Japan, situated along the Pacific Ring of Fire, is blessed with abundant geothermal activity. *Onsen*, sourced from these natural hot springs, are considered gifts from the *kami*, Shinto deities believed to inhabit natural elements. The sacred nature of the *onsen* is ingrained in the Japanese cultural psyche.

Purity and Rituals:
Entering an *onsen* is not merely a matter of hygiene; it is a ritualized practice rooted in notions of purity. Before stepping into the communal bath, individuals are expected to thoroughly cleanse themselves, both symbolically and physically, at washstations. This purification ritual reflects the Shinto concept of tsumi, or impurity, and prepares bathers for the sacred experience.

Seasonal Significance:
Onsen bathing is a dynamic practice influenced by the changing seasons. The Japanese deeply appreciate the beauty of nature, and *onsen* experiences vary with the seasons. Bathing in the outdoor *rotenburo* during a snowfall or enjoying the cherry blossoms in spring enhances the spiritual connection with the natural world.

Spiritual Cleansing and Mindfulness:
The act of bathing in an *onsen* extends beyond the physical; it is a form of spiritual cleansing. Immersed in the warm waters, surrounded by nature, bathers often engage in mindfulness. The meditative quality of the *onsen* experience fosters a sense of tranquility and encourages contemplation.

Respect for Nature:
Japanese *onsen* culture emphasizes respect for nature. The siting of *onsen* in scenic landscapes, often with views of mountains, forests, or the sea, is intentional. The integration of the *onsen* with nature is believed to enhance the therapeutic and spiritual benefits of the experience.

Community and Social Harmony:
While *onsen* bathing is often a solitary experience, communal bathing fosters a sense of social harmony. The shared space becomes a venue for quiet camaraderie, where individuals, stripped of societal roles, connect on a more authentic level. The egalitarian nature of the *onsen* promotes a communal sense of well-being.

The traditional Chinese steam baths and Japanese *onsen* exemplify the Far East's nuanced approach to bathing, incorporating philosophies of balance, spirituality, and connection with nature. From the harmonizing principles of Traditional Chinese Medicine to the sacred purity rituals of Japanese *onsen*, these practices reflect a profound understanding of the interplay between physical and spiritual well-being in Far Eastern cultures.

Indigenous Steam Practices: Native American Sweat Lodges

In the vast and diverse landscapes of North America, Native American cultures developed a unique practice of communal steam bathing known as sweat lodges. These structures, often woven into the fabric of tribal ceremonies, were more than places for physical cleansing; they were sacred spaces where spiritual purification, community bonding, and connection with the natural world converged.

Sacred Design and Rituals:
Sweat lodges were constructed with careful consideration of the surrounding environment and traditional beliefs. Typically made from natural materials such as willow branches and animal hides, these structures embodied a deep connection with the earth. Rituals associated with sweat lodges varied among tribes but often involved prayers, chanting, and the use of sacred herbs like sage and cedar to enhance the spiritual atmosphere.

Spiritual Purification:
The practice of entering a sweat lodge was seen as a journey of spiritual purification. The intense heat generated by hot stones, often infused with water and aromatic herbs, induced sweating, symbolizing the release of impurities from both the body and the spirit. The experience was not only physically challenging but also a profound form of introspection and connection with the sacred.

Community Bonding and Support:
Sweat lodges played a crucial role in fostering community bonding. Participants, regardless of age or status, shared the enclosed space, creating an egalitarian environment. The shared experience of the sweat lodge, with its physical and spiritual challenges, strengthened social ties and offered a sense of support within the tribal community.

Connection with the Natural World:
The construction of sweat lodges often involved a deep understanding of the natural world. The choice of materials, the orientation of the lodge, and the incorporation of natural elements in rituals reflected the indigenous peoples' profound connection with the land. Sweat lodge ceremonies were often aligned with celestial events or natural cycles, reinforcing the harmony between human life and the environment.

Indigenous Australian Steam Rituals

In the vast expanse of Australia, Indigenous cultures developed steam rituals that were integral to their connection with the land, spirituality, and the Dreamtime — the ancestral period of creation. These steam rituals, often associated with sacred sites and natural thermal springs, held profound significance in Indigenous Australian communities.

Sacred Sites and Dreamtime Connection:
Indigenous Australian steam rituals were intricately tied to sacred sites believed to be imbued with spiritual energy. These sites, often associated with Dreamtime stories, were considered portals to the spiritual realm. The use of steam in these rituals was seen as a means of communing with ancestral spirits and tapping into the Dreamtime narratives that shaped Indigenous cosmology.

Thermal Springs and Healing Traditions:
Natural thermal springs, scattered across the Australian landscape, were key locations for steam rituals. Indigenous communities believed in the healing properties of these thermal waters, seeing them as gifts from ancestral beings. The incorporation of steam in these rituals was not only for physical cleansing but also for invoking spiritual healing and balance.

Connection with Totemic Beings:
Indigenous Australian cultures often associated totemic beings with specific landscapes and features. Steam rituals were conducted in places where these totemic beings were believed to reside. The rising steam was seen as a manifestation of the presence of ancestral spirits, creating a bridge between the physical and spiritual realms.

Art and Symbolism:
Steam rituals were often accompanied by intricate body paintings and symbolic art. These visual elements played a role in expressing cultural identity, conveying Dreamtime stories, and invoking the energy of the land. The steam, rising in harmony with the artistry, became a visual representation of the spiritual interconnectedness between the people and the environment.

Sustainable Practices:
Indigenous Australian steam rituals exemplified a deep respect for the land and sustainable practices. The utilization of natural thermal springs and the careful observance of cultural protocols ensured that these rituals were in harmony with the ecological balance. Indigenous communities considered themselves custodians of the land, and steam rituals were conducted with a sense of responsibility towards the environment.

Indigenous steam practices in both Native American and Indigenous Australian cultures reflect a profound understanding of the interplay between physical and spiritual well-being. From the sweat lodges of North America, fostering community bonding and spiritual purification, to the steam rituals in Australia, deeply connected to Dreamtime narratives and healing traditions, these practices are testament to the rich cultural tapestry woven by indigenous communities across the globe.

Cross-Cultural Influences: Trade Routes and Exchange of Steam Practices

The intricate web of historical trade routes served as conduits not only for goods but also for the exchange of cultural practices. Steam, with its diverse applications in bathing rituals, became a shared cultural thread that traversed continents, fostering a cross-cultural exchange that transcended borders and enriched the practices of diverse societies.

Silk Road and the Flow of Ideas:
The Silk Road, a network of trade routes connecting East and West, was a melting pot of cultural exchange. As merchants traversed the vast expanse from China to the Mediterranean, they carried not only silk, spices, and precious goods but also the intangible wealth of ideas. Steam practices, including bathing traditions, were shared along this ancient route, influencing the wellness rituals of cultures from the Far East to the Middle East and Europe.

Spread of Bathhouses and *Hammams*:
The concept of communal bathing, often accompanied by steam rituals, spread along trade routes and found a home in diverse cultures. The *Hammams* of Babylon, influenced by Mesopotamian and Persian practices, became centers of communal life in the Middle East. Turkish *hammams*, with their own unique variations on steam bathing, evolved as prominent features in Ottoman culture, influenced by both Eastern and Western traditions.

Medieval European Influences:
In medieval Europe, where trade routes connected the East and the West, the exchange of ideas extended to bathing practices. The Crusaders returning from the Holy Land brought with them the influence of *hammams* and bathing rituals. European bathhouses, once simple structures, began to incorporate elements inspired by Eastern practices, transforming into spaces for social interaction and communal well-being.

Shared Symbolism in Steam Rituals

The symbolism associated with steam rituals transcends geographical boundaries, creating a universal language that communicates themes of purification, renewal, and spiritual ascent. Across cultures, the rising steam became a metaphorical bridge connecting the physical and metaphysical realms, embodying shared human experiences and aspirations.

Purification and Renewal:
One of the common threads in steam rituals is the symbolism of purification. Whether in the sweat lodges of Native American cultures, the Japanese *onsen*, or the Roman *thermae*, the act of bathing in steam was associated with cleansing the body and spirit. The rising steam was believed to carry away impurities, allowing individuals to emerge renewed and revitalized.

Connection with the Divine:
Steam rituals often incorporated elements of spiritual connection. In *Hammams* of Babylon, prayers were offered during bathing, connecting the act to religious devotion. Japanese *onsen* bathing, with its emphasis on purity, reflects Shinto beliefs in connecting with the *kami*, spiritual beings associated with nature. The rising steam became a conduit for communing with the divine in various cultural contexts.

Symbolism of Transformation:
The transformative power of steam, symbolizing change and metamorphosis, resonated across cultures. In Chinese steam baths, the warming properties of steam aligned with concepts of balance and transformation in Traditional Chinese Medicine. Similarly, the sweat lodges of Native American cultures were spaces where the intense heat symbolized not just physical release but a spiritual metamorphosis.

Communal Harmony:
The communal aspect of steam rituals, where individuals come together in shared spaces, signifies a universal longing for communal harmony. Whether in the Roman *thermae*, Turkish *hammams*, or Indigenous Australian steam rituals, the shared experience of bathing fosters a sense of community, breaking down societal barriers and fostering a collective sense of well-being.

Environmental Connection:
Steam rituals often reflect a deep connection with the natural environment. Indigenous practices, such as those in Native American sweat lodges or Indigenous Australian steam rituals, involve a symbiotic relationship with the land. The rising

steam becomes a symbolic bridge between the human community and the natural world, reinforcing a sense of interconnectedness.

The exchange of steam practices along historical trade routes and the shared symbolism in steam rituals reveal the interconnectedness of human cultures. Whether in the Far East, the Middle East, Europe, or the Americas, the rising steam serves as a universal language, communicating themes of purification, renewal, and communal harmony that transcend cultural boundaries and enrich the tapestry of human experience.

Common Elements Across Ancient Cultures: Purification and Ritualistic Cleansing

Across diverse ancient cultures, a common thread weaves through the fabric of communal bathing practices – the profound significance of purification and ritualistic cleansing. Whether in the sweat lodges of Native American cultures, the *Hammams* of Babylon, or the Roman *thermae*, the act of bathing in steam transcended mere physical cleanliness to become a sacred ritual with deep spiritual and symbolic implications.

Symbolism of Renewal:
Purification through steam bathing symbolized a process of renewal. The rising steam, enveloping the bather, carried away not only physical impurities but also metaphorical burdens and stresses. This symbolic cleansing represented a rebirth, a shedding of the old to make way for the new.

Spiritual Purity:
The act of ritualistic cleansing in steam was closely tied to achieving spiritual purity. In Native American sweat lodges, the intense heat represented a spiritual challenge, a means of purifying both the body and the spirit. Similarly, in the *Hammams* of Babylon or Roman *thermae*, bathing was imbued with spiritual significance, aligning with the cultural beliefs of the time.

Connection with Deities:
In many ancient cultures, steam rituals involved a connection with deities or divine forces. Prayers and invocations often accompanied the bathing process, seeking favor from gods associated with water and purification. The rising steam became a conduit for communication with the divine, forging a link between the earthly and the spiritual realms.

Cultural Symbolism:
The symbolism of purification through steam was deeply ingrained in cultural practices. Whether guided by the principles of Traditional Chinese Medicine, where steam baths aimed to balance the body's vital forces, or influenced by Roman concepts of hygiene and communal well-being, the cultural symbolism surrounding purification rituals reflected the values and beliefs of each society.

Common Elements Across Ancient Cultures: Spiritual and Therapeutic Dimensions of Steam

Beyond the physical act of cleansing, the use of steam in ancient cultures carried profound spiritual and therapeutic dimensions. The rising vapors were not only a means of achieving bodily health but also a conduit for spiritual connection and holistic well-being.

Spiritual Ascent:
Steam rituals often symbolized a spiritual ascent, a journey towards higher consciousness or divine connection. In the Japanese *onsen*, the act of immersing oneself in the warm waters amid natural surroundings became a form of spiritual cleansing and alignment with the sacred. The rising steam contributed to the meditative quality of the experience.

Therapeutic Benefits:
Ancient cultures recognized the therapeutic properties of steam. From the Roman *thermae*, where individuals indulged in hot baths for relaxation and muscle relief, to the Chinese steam baths with their focus on meridian therapy, the use of steam was integral to maintaining physical health and well-being.

Integration of Nature:
The therapeutic and spiritual dimensions of steam often involved an integration of nature. Indigenous Australian steam rituals conducted at natural thermal springs and Roman *thermae* situated amidst scenic landscapes exemplify this connection. The steam rituals became harmonious dialogues with the natural world, fostering a sense of balance and vitality.

Social and Communal Harmony:
The use of steam in communal bathing practices fostered social and communal harmony. Whether in the Far East, where communal bathing in *onsen* became a shared cultural experience, or in the sweat lodges of Native American tribes, the act of bathing in steam was a communal endeavor that transcended individual boundaries, reinforcing social bonds and collective well-being.

Continuity in Modern Wellness:
The spiritual and therapeutic dimensions associated with steam in ancient cultures continue to influence modern wellness practices. Contemporary spa cultures, with their emphasis on relaxation, stress relief, and holistic well-being, owe a debt to the enduring legacy of the spiritual and therapeutic dimensions of steam from the ancient world.

The common elements of purification and ritualistic cleansing, as well as the spiritual and therapeutic dimensions of steam across ancient cultures, reveal a shared human understanding of the profound connection between the physical, spiritual, and communal aspects of well-being. These ancient practices continue to resonate in contemporary wellness, demonstrating the enduring relevance of the rituals that transcend time and cultural boundaries.

Legacy and Influence: How Ancient Steam Rituals Shape Modern Wellness

The legacy of ancient steam rituals resonates through time, shaping and influencing modern wellness practices. From the sweat lodges of Native American cultures to the Roman *thermae* and Japanese *onsen*, the enduring impact of these ancient traditions is evident in contemporary spa cultures, holistic wellness approaches, and a growing appreciation for the interconnectedness of physical, spiritual, and communal well-being.

Contemporary Spa Culture:
Modern spa culture owes much to the ancient steam rituals that prioritized relaxation, purification, and holistic well-being. Spa experiences worldwide draw inspiration from the communal bathing practices of ancient civilizations, offering steam rooms, hot baths, and saunas as integral components of therapeutic and rejuvenating treatments.

Stress Relief and Relaxation:
The therapeutic dimensions associated with steam in ancient cultures, such as the Roman *thermae*, have found resonance in contemporary stress relief practices. Steam rooms and saunas are now recognized for their ability to promote relaxation, alleviate muscle tension, and provide a sanctuary for mental rejuvenation. The meditative quality of these spaces reflects a continuity from ancient spiritual dimensions.

Holistic Wellness:
The holistic approach to wellness embedded in ancient steam rituals has shaped modern perceptions of well-being. The integration of physical, spiritual,

and communal aspects is evident in wellness retreats, where practices like meditation, yoga, and communal bathing experiences draw inspiration from the comprehensive approach to health seen in ancient cultures.

Thermal Bath Tourism:
Ancient practices, particularly those associated with thermal baths, have fueled a resurgence in thermal bath tourism. The popularity of visiting natural hot springs, modeled after traditions like the Japanese *onsen* and Indigenous Australian steam rituals, reflects a growing interest in the therapeutic benefits of natural thermal waters.

Influence on Architectural Design:
The architectural design of modern spa facilities often echoes the grandeur of ancient bathhouses. Elements inspired by the Hammams of Babylon, Roman *thermae*, and Far Eastern bathing traditions are incorporated into contemporary structures, creating spaces that seamlessly blend historical aesthetics with modern functionality.

Preservation of Cultural Steam Practices

Preserving cultural steam practices is crucial for maintaining the authenticity and richness of diverse traditions. Efforts to safeguard and transmit these practices to future generations involve a balance between conservation, education, and cultural appreciation.

Cultural Heritage Initiatives:
Numerous cultural heritage initiatives focus on preserving and promoting traditional steam practices. Efforts include the documentation of rituals, the restoration of ancient bathing structures, and educational programs that raise awareness about the cultural significance of steam rituals.

Intergenerational Transmission:
Preservation involves passing down knowledge and practices from one generation to the next. In communities where steam rituals are integral to cultural identity, efforts are made to ensure that younger generations are actively involved in and informed about these practices, fostering a sense of continuity.

Collaboration with Indigenous Communities:
In regions with Indigenous steam rituals, collaborative initiatives with Indigenous communities are vital. These collaborations prioritize the insights and expertise of the communities themselves, ensuring that preservation efforts are culturally sensitive and align with the values and perspectives of the people involved.

Sustainable Practices:
Preservation efforts also consider the environmental impact of steam rituals. Sustainable practices, such as the responsible use of natural thermal springs and the incorporation of eco-friendly technologies in steam facilities, contribute to the long-term preservation of both cultural practices and the natural environment.

Global Recognition and Appreciation:
The recognition of cultural steam practices on a global scale fosters appreciation and understanding. Cultural exchange programs, festivals, and educational initiatives contribute to a broader awareness of the significance of steam rituals, fostering cross-cultural appreciation and respect.

The legacy of ancient steam rituals is not only evident in the shaping of modern wellness practices but also in the ongoing efforts to preserve and celebrate cultural traditions. As we navigate the contemporary landscape of spa cultures and holistic wellness, the influence of ancient steam rituals serves as a testament to the enduring wisdom embedded in these age-old practices. The preservation of cultural steam rituals ensures that these rich traditions continue to enrich the global tapestry of human well-being.

Evolution of Steam Practices in Medieval Times: Transition from Ancient to Medieval Steam Practices

The transition from ancient to medieval times marked a period of dynamic cultural and societal shifts, influencing various aspects of life, including bathing and steam practices. While certain continuity existed from antiquity, medieval steam practices underwent transformations shaped by the convergence of cultural, religious, and medical influences.

Continuity from Antiquity:
The Roman Empire's decline and the onset of the medieval period did not lead to an abrupt departure from ancient steam practices. In regions where Roman influence persisted, public baths and bathing traditions endured, albeit with changes influenced by the evolving socio-political landscape.

Christianization and Cultural Shifts:
The spread of Christianity across Europe during the medieval period brought about changes in societal norms and cultural practices. The Roman *thermae*, once vibrant communal spaces, faced challenges as Christian moralists expressed reservations about public nudity and mixed-gender bathing. Consequently, bathhouses became more modest and private.

Influence of Islamic Bathing Traditions:
In regions where Islamic influence extended, such as the Iberian Peninsula, Islamic bathing traditions, particularly the *Hammams,* left a lasting impact. The intricate design and architectural elements of *Hammams* influenced the development of bathhouses in medieval Europe.

Medical Theories and Balneology:
Medieval steam practices were significantly influenced by prevailing medical theories. During this time, the study of balneology, the therapeutic use of bathing, gained prominence. Medical treatises, like those of medieval physicians Avicenna and Trotula, advocated for the therapeutic benefits of bathing in hot water, emphasizing its role in promoting health and treating various ailments.

Four Humors and Balancing the Body:
Medieval medical theories were often grounded in the concept of the four humors—blood, phlegm, black bile, and yellow bile. Balneology in the medieval period emphasized the need to balance these humors for optimal health. Steam baths were recommended as a means to open the pores, induce sweating, and expel excess humors, aligning with the broader goal of restoring bodily equilibrium.

Emergence of Spa Towns:
The medieval period saw the emergence of spa towns and resorts, where natural hot springs were harnessed for therapeutic purposes. These locations became centers for balneology, attracting individuals seeking remedies for various ailments. The development of spa towns signaled a shift towards more intentional and specialized approaches to bathing.

Symbolism and Cultural Practices:
Medieval steam practices continued to carry symbolic and cultural significance. Bathing, often associated with notions of cleanliness, purity, and spiritual well-being, retained ritualistic elements. Despite variations in practices across regions, the act of bathing retained its importance in both personal hygiene and societal norms.

Challenges and Contrasts:
The medieval period presented challenges and contrasts in steam practices. While some regions embraced bathing for its therapeutic and hygienic benefits, others faced periods of decline in bathing culture, influenced by socio-religious factors and economic challenges.

The evolution of steam practices in medieval times reflected a nuanced interplay of continuity from ancient traditions, religious influences, medical theories, and cultural shifts. The transition marked both preservation and transformation, laying the groundwork for the diverse bathing practices that would emerge in subsequent historical periods. The medieval period, with its dynamic blend of influences, played a pivotal role in shaping the trajectory of steam practices in the Western world.

Steam & Bathing in The Renaissance

While the Renaissance did not witness the full realization of steam engines and steam technology as we know them today, it played a crucial role in laying the groundwork for steam technology. Additionally, the era saw a renewed interest in thermal bathing and the potential health benefits of steam, setting the stage for the later development of steam-based therapies and the integration of steam into medical practices during subsequent historical periods.

Thermal Bathing and Health: The Renaissance saw a resurgence of interest in thermal bathing and its potential health benefits. Spa towns, often centered around natural hot springs, gained popularity. The use of hot baths was believed to have therapeutic effects on various ailments, although the understanding of these effects was often based on traditional and sometimes mystical beliefs.

Hydrotherapy and Balneology: The Renaissance witnessed a revival of interest in hydrotherapy and balneology—the therapeutic use of bathing. Physicians began to recommend specific bathing practices for various conditions, aligning with the Renaissance emphasis on empirical observation and experimentation.

Influence of Ancient Medical Texts: Renaissance scholars revisited ancient medical texts, including those from Greco-Roman and Islamic traditions. These texts often contained references to bathing and the use of steam for health purposes. Renaissance physicians sought inspiration from these classical sources while integrating emerging scientific principles.

Emergence of Spas as Health Resorts: Spa towns, with their natural thermal springs, became popular destinations for those seeking health and wellness. The Renaissance saw the establishment of spa resorts that offered a range of bathing experiences, including hot baths, saunas, and steam rooms, often associated with medicinal properties. Examples include:

- **Montecatini Terme**, located in Tuscany, Italy, is one of the most famous spa towns with a history dating back to the 14th century. However, it gained prominence during the Renaissance when the Medici family recognized its therapeutic properties.

  The town is known for its thermal waters, and various spas and bathhouses were established to cater to visitors seeking the health benefits of the natural springs.

- **Bagni di Pisa,** also known as San Giuliano Terme, is located near Pisa in Tuscany, Italy. It was known for its thermal baths and gained popularity during the Renaissance.

The Medici family played a role in developing the spa, and it became a destination for the European aristocracy seeking the purported health benefits of the thermal waters.

In a Renaissance thermal bath, a noble could expect:

1. **Balneotherapy:** Immersing in mineral-rich waters for relaxation and health benefits.

2. **Hydrotherapy:** Using water in various forms, like baths and showers, for therapeutic purposes.

3. **Drinking Mineral Waters:** Consuming mineral-rich water for internal health benefits.

4. **Massage and Manual Therapies:** Relaxing treatments to relieve tension and improve circulation.

5. **Exercise:** Engaging in physical activities for overall well-being.

6. **Herbal Remedies and Aromatherapy:** Using herbs and essential oils for therapeutic effects.

7. **Social Activities:** Participating in social and recreational events for mental well-being.

Symbolic Importance of Cleanliness: The Renaissance placed symbolic importance on cleanliness and personal hygiene. Bathing, including steam baths, became associated not only with physical health but also with moral and spiritual purity, reflecting broader cultural shifts during this period.

§

18th-Century Spa Culture: The Emergence of Health Resorts and Spa Towns

The 18th century witnessed a significant resurgence of interest in health and wellness, leading to the emergence of health resorts and spa towns across Europe. This period marked a cultural shift where individuals sought not only therapeutic treatments but also recreational and social experiences centered around water, bathing, and the healing properties of spa environments.

Health Resorts and Spa Towns:

1. Renewed Interest in Hydrotherapy: The 18th century saw a revival of interest in hydrotherapy, emphasizing the therapeutic benefits of water in various forms. Spa towns became popular destinations, offering a range of hydrotherapeutic treatments, including bathing in natural springs, hot baths, and other water-based therapies.

2. Role of Mineral Springs: Spa towns were often situated around natural mineral springs, believed to possess unique healing properties. The mineral content of these springs was thought to contribute to the therapeutic effects of the water, attracting visitors seeking relief from various ailments.

3. Cultural and Social Centers: Spa towns evolved into cultural and social hubs where individuals from different backgrounds converged. The allure of health, recreation, and social interaction made spa culture a significant aspect of 18th-century European society.

4. Architectural Developments: The popularity of spa culture led to the construction of grand architectural structures in spa towns. Elaborate bathhouses, pump rooms, and gardens were built to enhance the overall spa experience. These structures often reflected the architectural styles of the time, showcasing the elegance and sophistication associated with spa culture.

5. Therapeutic Approaches: The therapeutic approaches offered in spa towns ranged from hydrotherapy to diverse wellness treatments. Visitors partook in mineral water drinking, bathing in hot springs, and engaging in various spa rituals believed to promote health and well-being.

6. Medicalization of Spa Practices: The 18th century witnessed a medicalization of spa practices, with physicians prescribing specific treatments based on individual health conditions. The belief in the medicinal properties of spa waters and the overall spa environment contributed to the integration of spa therapies into medical practices.

7. Literary and Artistic Influence: Spa culture permeated literature and the arts during the 18th century. Writers and artists depicted the allure of spa towns in their works, contributing to the cultural fascination with health resorts. The depiction of spa culture in literature and art further fueled the popularity of these destinations.

The Popularity of Steam Bathing in 18th-Century Europe

The 18th-century spa culture, marked by the emergence of health resorts and the popularity of steam bathing, reflected a dynamic period of societal transformation. Spa towns not only provided therapeutic treatments but also became centers of cultural, social, and recreational activities, influencing the broader wellness landscape in Europe during this era. The integration of steam bathing into spa practices laid the groundwork for its continued significance in later centuries.

1. Expansion of Bathhouse Facilities: Bathhouses in spa towns expanded to include steam rooms and saunas alongside traditional bathing facilities. The popularity of steam bathing grew as individuals sought the perceived benefits of steam for relaxation, cleansing, and overall well-being.

2. Hydrothermal Treatments: The understanding of hydrothermal treatments, including steam bathing, became more sophisticated. Spa-goers embraced the idea that exposure to steam could enhance circulation, promote detoxification through sweating, and contribute to skin health.

3. Social and Recreational Aspects: Steam bathing in the 18th century was not only a therapeutic practice but also a social and recreational activity. Spa-goers engaged in communal steam sessions, fostering a sense of camaraderie and shared well-being.

4. Integration into Wellness Regimens: Steam bathing became an integral component of comprehensive wellness regimens promoted in spa towns. Visitors followed prescribed routines that often included a combination of mineral water consumption, various bathing experiences, and steam rituals.

5. Cultural Symbolism: Steam bathing carried cultural symbolism associated with purity and cleanliness. The act of steaming was not only seen as physically beneficial but also as a ritual of purification and relaxation, aligning with broader cultural values of the time.

6. Continued Architectural Innovation: Bathhouse architecture continued to evolve in response to the growing popularity of steam bathing. Facilities were designed to accommodate steam rooms, incorporating innovations to enhance the steam experience.

7. Influence on European Society: The popularity of steam bathing in spa culture contributed to the broader influence of wellness practices on European society. The emphasis on health, leisure, and social interaction in spa towns reflected changing attitudes toward well-being and the desire for a holistic approach to health.

Public Bathhouses in the 19th Century: Development of Public Bathhouses during the 19th Century

The development of public bathhouses in the 19th century was a multifaceted phenomenon, influenced by urbanization, social reform movements, and a growing awareness of the importance of public health. These bathhouses not only addressed the practical need for improved hygiene in crowded urban environments but also became symbols of social progress and the promotion of community well-being.

1. Urbanization and Industrialization: The 19th century witnessed rapid urbanization and industrialization, leading to crowded and often unsanitary living conditions in burgeoning cities. As a response to the need for improved hygiene, public bathhouses began to emerge in urban centers.

2. Municipal Initiatives: Municipal governments recognized the importance of public health and sanitation. In response, many cities took the initiative to establish public bathhouses as part of broader public health campaigns. These bathhouses aimed to provide access to clean and affordable bathing facilities for the general population.

3. Architectural Innovation: Public bathhouses in the 19th century underwent architectural innovations. While earlier bathhouses were often simple structures, the 19th century saw the construction of more elaborate and purpose-built bathhouses. These buildings were designed to accommodate a larger number of people and offer a range of bathing options, including hot baths, showers, and steam rooms.

4. Diverse Bathing Options: Public bathhouses of the 19th century offered a variety of bathing options to cater to different preferences and needs. Some facilities provided traditional tub baths, while others incorporated communal showers and steam rooms. The goal was to make hygiene accessible to individuals from various socio-economic backgrounds.

5. Public Accessibility: Public bathhouses aimed for inclusivity and accessibility. They were designed to serve diverse segments of the population, including the working class. Many bathhouses offered low-cost or even free bathing opportunities, ensuring that even those with limited financial means could access sanitary facilities.

6. Cultural and Social Changes: The development of public bathhouses reflected evolving cultural attitudes toward cleanliness and hygiene. The Victorian era, in particular, emphasized moral and physical cleanliness. Public bathhouses became spaces where individuals could adhere to societal standards of cleanliness while also enjoying the social aspects of communal bathing.

7. Hygiene Education: Public bathhouses in the 19th century often incorporated hygiene education programs. Attendants provided information on the importance of cleanliness, proper bathing practices, and general health and sanitation. This educational component aimed to empower individuals to take charge of their health and well-being.

Social Reform Movements and Public Health Initiatives

1. Public Health Movement: The 19th century saw the rise of public health movements, driven by concerns about urban living conditions, disease outbreaks, and the overall well-being of the population. Public bathhouses became integral to these movements, promoting hygiene as a means to prevent the spread of infectious diseases.

2. Sanitary Reformers: Sanitary reformers, influenced by figures like Edwin Chadwick, advocated for improvements in public health infrastructure. They emphasized the connection between poor sanitation and disease, leading to increased awareness and support for public bathhouses as essential components of sanitation efforts.

3. Social Reform and Philanthropy: Philanthropic individuals and organizations played a significant role in the establishment of public bathhouses. The belief that improved hygiene could contribute to societal well-being motivated philanthropists to invest in the construction and maintenance of these facilities.

4. Temperance Movement: The Temperance Movement, which advocated for abstinence from alcohol, intersected with public health initiatives. Public bathhouses were often associated with temperance societies, providing alternative recreational spaces that promoted health and cleanliness without the presence of alcohol.

5. Women's Health Advocacy: Women's health advocates in the 19th century recognized the importance of hygiene for women's well-being. Public bathhouses, with their emphasis on cleanliness and health education, became spaces where women could access sanitary facilities and receive health guidance.

6. Legislation and Regulation: As awareness of public health issues grew, governments began to enact legislation to regulate sanitation standards. Public bathhouses became subject to these regulations, ensuring that they met established health and hygiene standards.

7. Integration into Social Welfare Programs: Public bathhouses were integrated into broader social welfare programs aimed at improving the living conditions of the working class. These facilities were seen as essential components of efforts to uplift communities by providing access to basic hygiene.

§

3. Steam & Health

Steam Therapy in 20th-Century Medicine: Integration into Medical Treatments

The 20th century witnessed the integration of steam into various medical treatments, ranging from respiratory health to physical therapy and rehabilitation. As the understanding of hydrotherapy and the therapeutic benefits of steam evolved, healthcare professionals recognized the diverse applications of steam therapy in promoting overall health and well-being. Steam's role in respiratory health and physical therapy reflects its versatility as a therapeutic modality in modern medicine.

1. Resurgence of Hydrotherapy: The 20th century witnessed a resurgence of interest in hydrotherapy, including the therapeutic use of steam. Medical professionals increasingly recognized the benefits of water-based treatments for various health conditions, leading to the integration of steam into medical protocols.

2. Incorporation into Rehabilitation Programs: Steam therapy became a valuable component of rehabilitation programs, particularly for individuals recovering from injuries or surgeries. The moist heat from steam was found to aid in muscle relaxation, improve joint mobility, and accelerate the healing process, making it a beneficial adjunct to physical therapy.

3. Orthopedic Applications: Steam therapy found applications in orthopedics, where it was utilized to alleviate pain and stiffness associated with musculoskeletal conditions. Patients with arthritis, joint inflammation, or chronic pain often benefited from the soothing and loosening effects of steam on affected areas.

4. Wound Care: Steam was incorporated into wound care practices, especially for chronic wounds or ulcers. The gentle warmth and increased blood circulation facilitated the healing process, contributing to improved outcomes in wound management.

5. Pulmonary Rehabilitation: Steam inhalation became a common practice in the treatment of respiratory conditions. The moist air was believed to soothe irritated airways, assist in mucus clearance, and provide relief for individuals with conditions such as asthma, bronchitis, or chronic obstructive pulmonary disease

6. **Sauna Therapy:** Sauna bathing, a form of dry heat therapy, gained popularity in the 20th century for its potential cardiovascular and respiratory benefits. Saunas, often utilizing steam as part of the heating process, became integral to wellness practices, with some studies suggesting positive effects on blood pressure and lung function.

7. **Balneotherapy and Spa Medicine:** The 20th century saw the continued integration of steam into balneotherapy, a holistic approach to health that involves the use of bathing, including steam baths, as a therapeutic modality. Spa medicine embraced steam as part of comprehensive wellness programs, emphasizing its role in relaxation, stress reduction, and overall health promotion.

Steam's Role in Respiratory Health and Physical Therapy

1. **Respiratory Conditions:** Steam inhalation was widely used to alleviate symptoms associated with respiratory conditions. Patients with conditions like sinusitis, allergies, or chest congestion found relief through inhaling steam, which helped to moisturize the airways, reduce inflammation, and promote easier breathing.

2. **Asthma Management:** Steam therapy became part of asthma management strategies. Inhaling warm, moist air from steam was believed to help open airways, potentially easing symptoms for individuals with asthma. However, it's important to note that medical opinions on the efficacy of steam therapy in asthma have varied.

3. **Postoperative Care:** Steam was incorporated into postoperative care protocols, particularly in orthopedic and joint surgeries. Steam's ability to relax muscles and improve circulation contributed to enhanced recovery and reduced postoperative discomfort.

4. **Rheumatologic Conditions:** Individuals with rheumatologic conditions, such as rheumatoid arthritis or osteoarthritis, benefited from steam therapy. The heat and moisture from steam helped to reduce joint stiffness and improve range of motion, offering relief for those with chronic musculoskeletal conditions.

5. **Sports Rehabilitation:** Steam therapy became a common feature in sports rehabilitation settings. Athletes recovering from injuries or undergoing physical therapy often used steam as part of their recovery routine to enhance flexibility, reduce muscle tension, and promote overall recovery.

6. Chronic Pain Management: Steam baths were utilized in chronic pain management programs. The combination of heat and moisture was thought to have analgesic effects, providing relief for individuals dealing with chronic pain conditions such as fibromyalgia or lower back pain.

7. Stress Reduction and Relaxation: Beyond specific medical applications, steam therapy played a crucial role in stress reduction and relaxation. The calming effect of steam on the nervous system contributed to its integration into holistic wellness practices aimed at improving mental well-being.

Research and Developments: Scientific Studies on the Health Benefits of Steam

Scientific studies on the health benefits of steam have provided valuable insights into its diverse applications in medicine and wellness. Advances in understanding the physiological effects of steam, from respiratory health to stress reduction and beyond, continue to contribute to evidence-based approaches in utilizing steam therapy for various health conditions.

While it is outside the scope of this work to present a comprehensive overview of the scientific research related to steam and health, the following examples provide examples of relevant work and may assist in guiding further self-directed research.

1. Respiratory Health:
- Numerous studies have investigated the impact of steam inhalation on respiratory health. Research suggests that inhaling warm, moist air can help alleviate symptoms of respiratory conditions such as sinusitis, allergies, and bronchitis. Steam is believed to soothe irritated airways, thin mucus, and facilitate easier breathing. A sample citation:

"Steam Inhalation Therapy: Efficacy and Mechanism of Action"

Reference: Singh M, et al. (2014). Journal of Otolaryngology and Rhinology.

Summary: This study explores the efficacy and potential mechanisms of action of steam inhalation therapy. It discusses how steam inhalation may influence respiratory health and contribute to symptom relief in conditions such as sinusitis and bronchitis.

2. Asthma Management:
- Studies have explored the use of steam therapy in asthma management. While opinions on its efficacy vary, some research indicates that inhaling warm steam may have a bronchodilator effect, potentially aiding individuals with asthma in managing their symptoms.

"The effect of steam inhalation on nasal obstruction and lung function in patients with allergic rhinitis and asthma"

Reference: Erkul E, Cingi C. (2014). American Journal of Rhinology & Allergy.

Summary: This study investigated the impact of steam inhalation on nasal obstruction and lung function in individuals with allergic rhinitis and asthma. The results suggested that steam inhalation might provide some benefit in terms of improving nasal symptoms and lung function in these patients.

3. Sinus Relief:
- Scientific investigations have focused on the benefits of steam in relieving sinus congestion. Steam inhalation is thought to moisturize the nasal passages, reduce inflammation, and promote sinus drainage, providing relief for individuals with sinus-related issues.

"Steam Inhalation Therapy: A Systematic Review"

Reference: Patel ZM, et al. (2016). The Laryngoscope.

Summary: While this review was mentioned earlier, it provides a broader overview of steam inhalation therapy, including its potential benefits for respiratory conditions. While not specific to sinus relief, it discusses the general effects of steam inhalation on nasal congestion and related symptoms.

4. Musculoskeletal Conditions:
- Scientific studies have explored the use of steam in managing musculoskeletal conditions. Steam's heat is believed to have analgesic effects, promoting muscle relaxation and reducing stiffness. This has implications for conditions such as arthritis and postoperative rehabilitation.

"Superficial Heat for Musculoskeletal Pain"

Authors: French SD, Cameron M, Walker BF, Reggars, JW, Esterman AJ.

Journal: Cochrane Database of Systematic Reviews. 2006.

Summary: This Cochrane review evaluates the effectiveness of superficial heat (including heat pads, warm packs, and heat wraps) for relieving musculoskeletal pain. While it doesn't specifically focus on steam, it provides insights into the broader use of heat therapy.

5. Stress Reduction and Mental Well-Being:
- Research has examined the psychological and physiological effects of steam therapy on stress reduction. Steam baths, often associated with relaxation, have been studied for their potential to reduce stress hormones, promote relaxation, and contribute to overall mental well-being.

"Effects of regular sauna bathing on symptoms, fatigue and quality of life in patients with chronic fatigue syndrome: a randomized controlled trial"

Authors: Luttikhold J, Oosterveld FGM, Jong M, Jong MC, Eijsvogels TMH, Hopman MTE.

Journal: BMC Complementary Medicine and Therapies. 2020.

Summary: This randomized controlled trial investigates the effects of regular sauna bathing on symptoms, fatigue, and quality of life in patients with chronic fatigue syndrome. While the primary focus is not on mental health, it explores the broader impact on well-being.

6. Cardiovascular Health:
- It's essential to note that while studies may have explored certain aspects related to cardiovascular health, steam therapy is not a primary or widely recognized intervention for cardiovascular conditions. Cardiovascular health is typically managed through lifestyle modifications, medications, and other evidence-based interventions. However, this study is of some significant interest:

"Regular sauna bathing and the risk of stroke: Evidence from a cohort study of 1.6 million Finns"

Authors: Kunutsor SK, Laukkanen T, Laukkanen JA.
Journal: Neurology. 2018.

Summary: This study explores the association between regular sauna bathing and the risk of stroke. While it primarily addresses cardiovascular outcomes, it provides insights into the potential health benefits of sauna use, which may indirectly impact mental well-being.

7. Skin Health:
- Scientific studies have explored the impact of steam on skin health. Steam is believed to open pores, cleanse the skin, and improve blood flow, potentially contributing to a healthier complexion. This has implications for skincare and dermatological conditions.

"The Influence of Finnish Sauna Baths on Skin Physiology: Perspiration, Transepidermal Water Loss, pH, Capillary Blood Flow and Skin Temperature"

Authors: Teija Kivijärvi, Kaisa Hannele Laihia, Markku Santala, Timo Puijonpää, Aki Sinkko, Markku Sipi, Saku Ruohonen, Kirsi Lappalainen.

Journal: Acta Dermato-Venereologica. 2019.

Summary: This study examines the influence of Finnish sauna baths, which involve exposure to high temperatures and steam, on various skin physiology parameters, including perspiration, transepidermal water loss, pH, capillary blood flow, and skin temperature.

8. Hydration and Detoxification:
- Investigations into the hydration and detoxification effects of steam therapy have been conducted. Steam baths are thought to promote sweating, aiding in the elimination of toxins and contributing to overall hydration, though the extent of these effects may vary.

"The effect of sauna bathing on total body water"

Authors: Mero AA, Tornberg J, Mäntykoski M, Puurtinen R.

Journal: Sports Medicine - Open. 2015.

Summary: This study investigates the effect of sauna bathing on total body water. It examines the potential impact of sauna exposure on hydration status and certain physiological parameters.

Advances in Understanding the Physiological Effects of Steam

1. Thermoregulation Mechanisms:
- Advances in thermoregulation research have contributed to a deeper understanding of how the body responds to heat, such as that provided by steam. This includes insights into the mechanisms underlying the dilation of blood vessels, increased heart rate, and sweating in response to heat exposure.

2. Neurological Responses:
- Neuroscientific studies have explored the neurological responses to steam therapy. The impact of steam on the central nervous system, including the release of neurotransmitters and endorphins, has been investigated to better comprehend the mechanisms behind the relaxing and stress-reducing effects of steam.

3. Inflammatory Pathways:
- Research has focused on the inflammatory pathways influenced by steam. Understanding how steam may modulate inflammation has implications for conditions where inflammation plays a role, such as in musculoskeletal disorders and wound healing.

4. Impact on Blood Flow and Circulation:
- Advances in vascular physiology have contributed to the understanding of how steam affects blood flow and circulation. Studies explore the vasodilatory effects of steam, which may lead to improved blood circulation and potential benefits for cardiovascular health.

5. Metabolic Effects:
- Scientific investigations have delved into the metabolic effects of steam therapy. This includes research on how exposure to heat, such as in a steam room, may influence metabolic rate, energy expenditure, and other metabolic processes.

6. Hydration Dynamics:
- Advances in hydration science have contributed to understanding the dynamics of hydration in steam therapy. Research examines how steam-induced sweating contributes to fluid balance and detoxification processes in the body.

7. Genetic and Molecular Responses:
- Molecular studies have explored the genetic and molecular responses to steam exposure. This includes investigating changes in gene expression and molecular pathways associated with the physiological effects of steam on various body systems.

8. Psychoneuroimmunology of Relaxation:
- Integrating findings from psychoneuroimmunology, researchers have explored the connections between mental relaxation induced by steam therapy, neurological responses, and the modulation of the immune system. This interdisciplinary approach contributes to a holistic understanding of the physiological effects of steam on overall well-being.

Psychoneuroimmunology

Psychoneuroimmunology (PNI) is an interdisciplinary field that explores the intricate connections between the nervous system, the endocrine system, and the immune system. The term itself reflects the integration of three major systems: psycho (involving psychological factors), neuro (referring to the nervous system), and immunology (related to the immune system).

Key Components of Psychoneuroimmunology

1. Psychological Factors: PNI investigates how psychological factors, such as stress, emotions, cognition, and behavior, can influence the immune system. Stress, for example, has been shown to impact immune function, and PNI seeks to understand the underlying mechanisms.

2. Nervous System: The nervous system, comprising the central nervous system (brain and spinal cord) and the peripheral nervous system, communicates with the immune system through neural pathways. Neurotransmitters and neuropeptides released by nerve cells can influence immune responses.

3. Endocrine System: Hormones produced by the endocrine system, particularly the hypothalamus, pituitary gland, and adrenal glands (the HPA axis), play a crucial role in the regulation of immune function. PNI examines how hormonal signals impact immune cells and responses.

4. Immune System: The immune system is responsible for defending the body against pathogens and maintaining overall health. PNI studies how psychological and neurological factors can modulate immune function, affecting aspects such as inflammation, immune cell activity, and antibody production.

Research Areas in Psychoneuroimmunology

1. Stress and Immune Function: PNI research has extensively explored the impact of stress on the immune system. Chronic stress, for instance, has been associated with alterations in immune responses and increased susceptibility to illness.

2. Emotions and Immune Responses: Studies examine how emotions, such as happiness, sadness, and anxiety, can influence immune function. Positive emotions are often correlated with better immune outcomes.

3. Cognitive Processes: PNI investigates how cognitive processes, including beliefs, attitudes, and perceptions, can affect immune responses. The field explores the concept of psychosocial factors influencing health outcomes.

4. Mind-Body Interventions: Research in PNI includes the study of mind-body interventions, such as meditation, mindfulness, and relaxation techniques, and their potential effects on immune function and overall health.

5. Neurotransmitters and Immune Modulation: PNI delves into the role of neurotransmitters, such as serotonin and dopamine, in influencing immune cells and responses.

Clinical Implications:
Understanding the interactions between psychological, neurological, and immunological factors has implications for health and disease. PNI research may contribute to the development of interventions that promote overall well-being, manage stress-related disorders, and enhance immune function.

Relevance to Steam and Sauna

The field of psychoneuroimmunology (PNI) has relevance to the context of steam and sauna use, particularly in how these heat-based therapies may impact the interconnected systems of the body.

1. Stress Reduction: Steam and sauna sessions are often associated with relaxation and stress reduction. PNI studies have shown that chronic stress can have negative effects on the immune system. Therefore, activities that help reduce stress, such as sauna sessions, may indirectly contribute to maintaining a healthier immune function.

2. Neurotransmitter Release: Heat exposure in saunas can stimulate the release of neurotransmitters, including endorphins. Endorphins are known for their role in promoting a sense of well-being. PNI explores how such neurotransmitters can influence both the nervous and immune systems.

3. Hormonal Regulation: Sauna use can lead to changes in hormone levels, including those related to the stress response (e.g., cortisol). PNI investigates how these hormonal changes may impact immune function and overall health.

4. Immune Modulation: While the immediate impact of sauna use on the immune system is often temporary, regular sessions may have long-term effects on immune function. PNI research explores how various interventions, including stress reduction strategies, can modulate immune responses over time.

5. Mind-Body Connection: Sauna and steam practices involve a mind-body connection, where the perception of warmth and relaxation can influence both psychological and physiological responses. PNI examines how the mind and body interact and how mental states can influence immune function.

6. Inflammation and Heat Therapy: Some PNI studies explore the relationship between inflammatory processes in the body and interventions like heat therapy. Sauna use has been suggested as a potential way to modulate inflammation, and PNI may provide insights into the underlying mechanisms.

It's important to note that while sauna and steam practices may have potential benefits for stress reduction and overall well-being, the specific impact on immune function can vary among individuals. Additionally, the existing research may not exclusively focus on sauna or steam treatments but rather on the broader concepts of heat therapy and stress reduction.

Individuals considering sauna or steam sessions as part of their wellness routine should approach these practices as complementary to an overall healthy lifestyle, including regular exercise, a balanced diet, and adequate hydration. As with any health-related practices, consulting with healthcare professionals is advisable, especially for individuals with pre-existing health conditions.

4. Detoxification, Steam & Sweating Safely

Detoxification refers to the process of removing toxins from the body to improve health. It encompasses a range of interventions aimed at managing acute intoxication and withdrawal, with the primary goal of minimizing the physical harm caused by the abuse of substances, or ingestion of substances through environment, foods or water that could be harmful to the normal processes and healthy operations of the body.

Types of Detoxification

1. Medical Detoxification: This involves the use of physician and nursing staff, along with medication, to assist individuals through withdrawal safely.

2. Full-Body Detox: This typically involves following a specific diet or using special products to rid the body of toxins, with the aim of improving health and promoting weight loss.

Methods of Detoxification

1. Sweating: Regular sweating through exercise, sauna sessions, or steam rooms is considered a method of detoxification.

2. Medically Assisted Detox: This form of detox is supported by trained specialists and aims to minimize the negative impact of withdrawal symptoms, from chemical addictions, making the experience as safe and comfortable as possible.

Misconceptions and Considerations

Detox diets and products are often marketed as ways to eliminate toxins from the body, but it's important to note that the body naturally eliminates harmful substances without requiring special diets or supplements. Sweating is one method the body uses for this process.

Sweating Safely

Sweating, facilitated by steam therapy, is considered a safe and effective way to aid the body in the detoxification process and improve overall health.

Sweating is considered a safe and effective way to assist in a detox regimen and improve health. Steam therapy, such as steam showers and steam rooms, can aid in the detoxification process by encouraging sweating, which allows the body to expel toxins through the skin. Steam showers are believed to be great for skin detoxes, as they encourage sweat and some toxins to naturally exit the body through the pores.

Additionally, a 10-15-minute steam session has been shown to help the body flush out potentially dangerous chemical irritants, and heavy metals were found to be excreted in sweat in greater quantities than urine.

All sweating practices should be acknowledged to provide support for the body's own sophisticated mechanisms for detoxification, primarily carried out by the liver and kidneys. These organs play a crucial role in processing and eliminating toxins from the body.
Sweating is a part of the body's temperature regulation system and contributes to fluid and electrolyte balance but is not the primary means of detoxification.

That being said, according to a study published in the Journal of Family Medicine and Community Health at the University of Wisconsin-Madison, sweating regularly through exercise, a sauna, or a steam room is considered a part of a good detox program.

Additionally, a review published in the National Center for Biotechnology Information suggests that normal sweating removes waste products and toxins from the body and is associated with maintaining good health.

5. Steam Best Practices

Incorporating steam into your home spa

can enhance relaxation, promote skin health, and contribute to an overall sense of well-being. Here are various methods you can consider:

1. Steam Shower:
   - Install a steam generator in your shower to create a dedicated steam shower space. Steam showers are designed with a steam-tight enclosure and a generator that releases steam into the sealed space, providing a convenient and enclosed environment for steam therapy.

2. Steam Sauna Room:
   - Designate a specific room or part of your bathroom as a steam sauna room.

You can achieve this by installing a steam generator and creating a well-sealed space. Ensure proper ventilation and consider adding comfortable seating for a more spa-like experience.

3. Steam Capsule or Pod:
- Explore steam capsules or pods designed for home use. These compact units are often easy to install and can be placed in existing bathrooms. They provide a private space for steam sessions without the need for major renovations.

4. Portable Steam Tent:
- Consider a portable steam tent that can be set up in various areas of your home. These tents typically include a steam generator and are designed to be easily assembled and disassembled. This option provides flexibility in choosing where to enjoy your steam sessions.

5. Steam Bath Generator:
- Install a steam bath generator in your existing shower or bathtub. This is a cost-effective way to add steam functionality to your current setup. Generators are available in various sizes to accommodate different space requirements.

6. DIY Steam Facial:
- Create a DIY steam facial by bringing steam to your face. Boil water and transfer it to a bowl, adding essential oils or herbs if desired. Lean over the bowl, covering your head with a towel to trap the steam. This method is suitable for a quick and simple steam experience.

7. Steam Inhalation Device:
- Use a steam inhalation device designed for home use. These devices often come with attachments for facial steaming or inhaling steam for respiratory benefits. They are portable and easy to use.

8. Steam Foot Bath:
- Enjoy a steam foot bath by placing a bowl of hot water infused with herbs or essential oils at your feet. Drape a towel over your head to create a mini steam experience while you soak your feet. This is a relaxing way to incorporate steam into your routine.

9. Aromatherapy Steam Diffusers:
- Integrate aromatherapy with steam by using essential oil diffusers designed for steam showers or sauna rooms. These devices disperse essential oil-infused steam, enhancing the sensory experience and providing additional therapeutic benefits.

10. Steam-Ready Bathtub:
   - Invest in a bathtub with steam capabilities. Some bathtubs come equipped with built-in steam generators, allowing you to enjoy the benefits of steam while soaking in a warm bath.

Remember to consider ventilation, safety measures, and the specific requirements of each method when incorporating steam into your home spa. Whether you choose a dedicated steam room or opt for smaller, portable solutions, creating a steam-enhanced environment can contribute to a luxurious and rejuvenating home spa experience.

Disclaimers & Important Points to Consider re: Steam Practices

The information provided here regarding steam therapy and its potential effects on health is intended for general informational purposes only. It is not a substitute for professional medical advice, diagnosis, or treatment. Before initiating any new health practices, including steam therapy, individuals are strongly advised to consult with qualified healthcare professionals.

That being said- Important Points to Consider:

1. Hydration: Steam therapy can induce sweating, leading to fluid loss. It is imperative to stay adequately hydrated by drinking sufficient water to replenish lost fluids.

2. Healthy Diet: Steam therapy should be complemented with a well-balanced and nutritious diet. Nutrient-rich foods contribute to overall health and support the body's various functions.

3. Exercise: Physical activity is a key component of a healthy lifestyle. Incorporating regular exercise into your routine can have numerous benefits for cardiovascular health, muscle strength, and overall well-being.

4. Weight Management: Maintaining a healthy weight is essential for overall health. It involves a combination of a balanced diet, regular exercise, and lifestyle choices.

5. Individual Variation: Responses to steam therapy and other wellness practices may vary among individuals. Factors such as pre-existing health conditions, medications, and individual sensitivities should be taken into consideration.

6. Consultation with Healthcare Professionals: Individuals with existing health conditions or those taking medications should seek guidance from healthcare professionals before incorporating new practices into their routine.

7. Holistic Well-Being: Health is a multifaceted concept that encompasses various aspects of physical, mental, and emotional well-being. Steam therapy should be viewed as one component of a larger, comprehensive approach to personal health.

Remember, everyone's health needs are unique, and individualized guidance from healthcare professionals is essential. This disclaimer serves as a general guide, and specific recommendations should be tailored to an individual's health status and requirements.

Cautions Related to Steam:

1. Pre-existing Health Conditions:
- Individuals with pre-existing health conditions such as cardiovascular issues, respiratory problems, or skin conditions should consult with a healthcare professional before engaging in steam sessions.

2. Pregnancy:
- Pregnant women should seek medical advice before using steam rooms or saunas, as excessive heat can pose risks to the developing fetus.

3. Hydration:
- It's essential to stay well-hydrated before entering a steam room to prevent dehydration, especially since steam induces sweating.

4. Duration of Sessions:
- Prolonged exposure to steam can lead to dehydration and overheating. Limit steam sessions to recommended durations and take breaks as needed.

5. Alcohol and Medications:
- Avoid consuming alcohol or taking medications that may impair your ability to regulate body temperature before entering a steam room.

6. Heat Sensitivity:
- Individuals sensitive to heat or prone to heat-related issues should exercise caution and consult with a healthcare professional before using steam facilities.

Best Practices Pre-Steam:

1. Hydration:
- Drink water before entering a steam room to ensure adequate hydration during the session.

2. Attire:
- Wear a swimsuit or comfortable clothing to allow your body to sweat freely. Remove any metal jewelry to prevent burns.

3. Skin Care:
- Remove makeup, lotions, or oils from your skin before entering the steam room to facilitate better absorption of steam.

4. Empty Stomach:
- Avoid heavy meals before a steam session to prevent discomfort and nausea.

5. Warm-up:
- Engage in light stretching or warm-up exercises to prepare your body for the heat.

Best Practices During Steam:

1. Duration:
- Limit steam sessions to 15-20 minutes or follow facility recommendations to avoid dehydration and overheating.

2. Seating:
- Sit or lie down to avoid dizziness. Use a towel on seating surfaces for hygiene.

3. Breathing:
- Breathe deeply and slowly to maximize the respiratory benefits of steam. Avoid shallow breathing.

4. Cool Down:
- Take breaks outside the steam room to cool down and rehydrate if needed.

Best Practices After Steam:

1. Hydration:
- Drink water to rehydrate after the steam session.

2. Cool Shower:
- Take a cool shower to bring your body temperature back to normal.

3. Rest:
- Allow time for rest and relaxation post-steam to maximize the benefits and prevent exhaustion.

4. Skincare:
- Moisturize your skin after the steam session to replenish lost moisture.

5. Recovery Period:
- Allow your body to recover before engaging in strenuous activities or additional heat exposure.

Remember, individual tolerance to steam varies, and it's crucial to listen to your body. If you experience dizziness, nausea, or discomfort, exit the steam room immediately and seek medical attention if necessary. Always follow the guidelines provided by the facility and consult with a healthcare professional if you have any health concerns.

Steam & Food

After a steam session, it's generally advisable to wait a short period before eating. This is because the heat from the steam can temporarily affect your digestive system, and eating immediately afterward may not be ideal. Here are some general recommendations:

1. Wait at Least 15-30 Minutes:
- Allow a brief cooling-down period after your steam session before consuming a meal. This gives your body time to return to its normal temperature and ensures that your digestive system is not overly stimulated.

2. Rehydrate First:
- Prioritize rehydration by drinking water after your steam session. This helps replenish fluids lost through sweating during the steam.

3. Listen to Your Body:
- Pay attention to how you feel. If you're hungry and feel comfortable, you can eat sooner. However, if you experience any discomfort, it's better to wait a bit longer.

4. Light, Nutrient-Rich Foods:
- When you decide to eat, opt for light and nutrient-rich foods. Fresh fruits, vegetables, lean proteins, and whole grains can be good choices to replenish nutrients without burdening your digestive system.

5. Avoid Heavy or Spicy Meals:
- Avoid heavy or spicy meals immediately after a steam session, as these can be harder on the digestive system. Opt for easily digestible foods to promote comfort.

6. Individual Variations:
- Individual reactions to steam sessions can vary. Some people may feel perfectly fine eating soon after, while others may prefer to wait a bit longer. Listen to your body's signals.

It's essential to note that these are general guidelines, and individual factors, such as your health condition and how your body responds to heat, can influence the timing. If you have any specific health concerns or conditions, it's advisable to consult with a healthcare professional for personalized advice.

6. STEAM TRAVEL

ICELAND.

Blue Lagoon, Iceland: A Geothermal Oasis Amidst Lava Fields

The Blue Lagoon in Iceland is more than a geothermal spa; it's a geological wonder, a cultural landmark, and a serene retreat where the warmth of the Earth's embrace meets the stark beauty of volcanic landscapes. As visitors soak in the mineral-rich waters and absorb the breathtaking surroundings, they become part of a narrative that transcends leisure—a story written by the Earth itself, inviting them to unwind in a place where the boundaries between nature and relaxation blur into a seamless, enchanting experience.

Nestled amidst the otherworldly landscapes of Iceland, the Blue Lagoon stands as an iconic geothermal oasis, drawing visitors from around the globe to indulge in the unique and rejuvenating experience it offers. With its mineral-rich waters and stunning surroundings, the Blue Lagoon is not just a destination; it's a natural masterpiece that harmonizes geothermal wonders with the rugged beauty of lava fields.

Mineral-Rich Geothermal Spa:

At the heart of the Blue Lagoon's allure lies its geothermal spa, a mesmerizing expanse of warm, mineral-rich waters. These milky-blue waters are not just visually stunning; they are infused with a unique blend of silica, algae, and minerals renowned for their skin-nourishing properties. Visitors immerse themselves in this geothermal embrace, surrendering to the soothing warmth that emanates from deep within the Earth.

Lava Fields Backdrop:

Surrounded by vast lava fields, the Blue Lagoon provides a surreal juxtaposition of elements. The stark, blackened terrain of ancient lava flows becomes a dramatic backdrop to the tranquil, azure waters. The contrast between the rugged lava formations and the serenity of the spa creates an otherworldly ambiance, inviting patrons to unwind in a setting that feels both primal and luxurious.

Natural Filtration Process:

The mineral-rich waters of the Blue Lagoon are not just a product of geological chance; they undergo a natural filtration process that takes place over an extended period. The water originates from the Svartsengi geothermal field, where it journeys through porous lava formations. Along the way, it picks up the unique blend of minerals that contribute to its therapeutic properties. This natural filtration process adds an authentic and organic dimension to the spa experience.

Skin-Healing Properties:

The silica-rich waters of the Blue Lagoon are believed to have exceptional skin-healing properties. Visitors often indulge in the ritual of applying silica mud masks, sourced directly from the lagoon, creating a spa experience that extends beyond mere relaxation. The minerals present in the water are said to promote skin health, leaving patrons with a radiant glow that reflects the natural benefits of the geothermal spa.

Year-Round Enchantment:

The Blue Lagoon's enchantment is not limited by the seasons; it offers a year-round retreat for visitors. In winter, guests can soak in the warm waters while surrounded by snow-covered lava fields, creating a magical contrast. In summer, the lagoon becomes a haven where the warmth of the water mingles with the endless daylight, providing a unique experience under the midnight sun.

Architectural Harmony:

The architecture of the Blue Lagoon complements the natural surroundings with a sense of contemporary elegance. Modern structures seamlessly blend with the landscape, providing amenities, changing facilities, and relaxation areas without compromising the integrity of the natural environment. The design ensures that visitors can enjoy the comforts of a world-class spa while remaining immersed in the unspoiled beauty of the Icelandic wilderness.

Cultural and Geological Significance:
Beyond its recreational appeal, the Blue Lagoon holds cultural and geological significance in Iceland. It symbolizes the country's commitment to sustainable geothermal practices and serves as a testament to the power of nature's therapeutic offerings. The lagoon has become an essential part of Iceland's identity, attracting visitors seeking both relaxation and a connection to the country's unique geological heritage.

SWITZERLAND.

Therme Vals, Switzerland: Architectural Marvel in Alpine Serenity

Nestled in the pristine Alpine landscapes of Switzerland, Therme Vals stands not just as a thermal spa but as an architectural masterpiece seamlessly integrated into the natural beauty that surrounds it. Designed by renowned architect Peter Zumthor, the spa offers visitors a unique blend of therapeutic relaxation and visual splendor, making it a destination that transcends the conventional spa experience.

Architectural Grandeur:
Therme Vals is an exemplar of architectural grandeur, showcasing Peter Zumthor's mastery in creating spaces that harmonize with their surroundings. The spa is crafted from locally quarried Valser Quartzite, a stone that not only lends a timeless aesthetic but also absorbs and reflects the changing light, allowing the building to merge organically with the Alpine environment. The architectural design itself becomes an integral part of the overall therapeutic experience.

Thermal Pools in Alpine Ambiance:
The thermal pools at Therme Vals are a celebration of the symbiosis between architecture and nature. The warm, mineral-rich waters of the pools invite visitors to immerse themselves in a serene aquatic experience, surrounded by the majestic Swiss Alps. Whether indoors or outdoors, the thermal pools become sanctuaries of relaxation where patrons can unwind while taking in the breathtaking Alpine vistas.

Natural Spring Water:
The therapeutic benefits of Therme Vals are rooted in the natural spring water that feeds the pools. Sourced from the Valser Valley, the water is rich in minerals with reputed healing properties. The journey of the water from its underground

origins to the pools is a testament to the spa's commitment to authenticity and the utilization of the region's natural resources.

Sculpted Light and Shadow:
One of the architectural marvels of Therme Vals is its manipulation of light and shadow. Large skylights, strategically placed windows, and carefully designed openings allow natural light to sculpt the interior spaces throughout the day. The interplay of light and shadow becomes a dynamic element, transforming the spa's ambiance and creating an ever-changing visual spectacle that enhances the sense of tranquility.

Sauna Suites as Sanctuaries:
Beyond the thermal pools, Therme Vals offers sauna suites as intimate sanctuaries of warmth and relaxation. The saunas are designed with meticulous attention to detail, incorporating the same Valser Quartzite to create a seamless connection with the overall architectural theme. Patrons can indulge in the therapeutic benefits of heat within spaces that echo the natural elegance of the surrounding landscape.

Integration with Nature:
Therme Vals is not just a structure placed in nature; it is a testament to the integration of architecture with its natural setting. Outdoor spaces, terraces, and pathways lead visitors through a journey where the boundaries between the spa and the Alpine environment blur. The design encourages a seamless transition from indoor to outdoor, allowing patrons to connect with nature at every turn.

Cultural and Wellness Retreat:
Therme Vals has become a cultural and wellness retreat that transcends the traditional spa experience. Beyond the physical relaxation, visitors are immersed in a sensory journey that engages sight, touch, and sound. The spa is not merely a destination; it's an escape that fosters a deep connection with the Swiss Alps, making it a cultural landmark that resonates with both locals and international visitors.

HUNGARY.

Gellért Baths, Hungary: Historic Elegance in Thermal Splendor

Situated in the heart of Budapest, the Gellért Baths are not merely a collection of pools but a testament to the rich thermal tradition of Hungary, housed within the iconic Gellért Hotel. Steeped in history and adorned with art nouveau elegance, these baths offer visitors a journey back in time while indulging in the therapeutic embrace of thermal waters.

Historic Significance:
The Gellért Baths boast a storied history that dates back to their opening in 1918. Built during the flourishing era of Art Nouveau, the baths have witnessed decades of social, cultural, and historical changes. The architecture itself is a nod to the grandeur of the past, providing patrons with a glimpse into a bygone era while offering a contemporary spa experience.

Art Nouveau Splendor:
The architectural charm of the Gellért Baths lies in their art nouveau splendor. Elaborate decorations, ornate details, and stained glass windows create an atmosphere of timeless elegance. The interplay of light within the intricately designed spaces adds a touch of sophistication, transforming the act of bathing into a refined and aesthetic experience.

Thermal Baths with Healing Waters:
At the heart of the Gellért Baths are the thermal pools, renowned for their healing properties. The thermal waters, sourced from the Gellért Hill's mineral-rich springs, are believed to have therapeutic benefits for various ailments. Visitors can immerse themselves in these revitalizing waters, surrounded by the architectural opulence that characterizes the baths.

Variety of Pools:
Gellért Baths offer a variety of pools catering to different preferences. From the thermal pools with their distinct temperatures to the swimming pool for those seeking exercise, patrons can tailor their experience to suit their needs. The Gellért Baths provide a space where the art of relaxation is harmoniously blended with options for recreation.

Outdoor Pool Oasis:
One of the highlights of the Gellért Baths is the outdoor pool oasis. Nestled within a courtyard surrounded by colonnades, the outdoor pool is a tranquil escape where visitors can enjoy the thermal waters amidst open skies. This al fresco setting adds a touch of natural serenity to the overall spa experience.

Architecture Meets Wellness:
The seamless integration of architectural grandeur with wellness is a defining feature of the Gellért Baths. The design pays homage to both form and function, ensuring that patrons not only benefit from the thermal waters but also revel in the immersive aesthetics that surround them. Each corner of the baths becomes a canvas where history, art, and wellness converge.

Cultural Hub:
The Gellért Baths have evolved into a cultural hub within Budapest. Beyond

their therapeutic offerings, the baths host events, concerts, and art exhibitions, fostering a vibrant atmosphere that resonates with locals and tourists alike. The cultural richness of the Gellért Baths extends beyond the pool waters, creating a space where wellness and the arts intertwine.

Iconic Status:
The Gellért Baths have achieved iconic status in Budapest, symbolizing the city's dedication to preserving its thermal heritage. Whether it's the striking facade of the building or the soothing waters within, the Gellért Baths have become a symbol of Budapest's commitment to maintaining its historic treasures while embracing modern wellness practices.

SPAIN.

Hammam Al Ándalus - Spain: A Journey into Andalusian Tranquility

Spanning the historic cities of Granada, Córdoba, and Málaga, Hammam Al Ándalus transports visitors into the heart of Andalusia's rich cultural heritage, offering a unique blend of traditional Arabic baths and historical spa indulgence. Each location becomes a gateway to a bygone era, where the ancient art of bathing is revived with elegance and authenticity.

Andalusian Architectural Splendor:
Hammam Al Ándalus is not just a spa; it's a testament to the architectural splendor of Andalusia. The moment visitors step into these baths, they are enveloped in the charm of Islamic-inspired design, characterized by intricately tiled mosaics, archways, and vaulted ceilings. The architecture pays homage to the region's historical connection to Al-Andalus, the medieval Muslim territory in the Iberian Peninsula.

Traditional Arabic Baths:
At the core of the Hammam Al Ándalus experience are the traditional Arabic baths. Divided into several rooms of varying temperatures, patrons embark on a circuit that includes hot, warm, and cold pools. The journey through these pools mimics the traditional Islamic approach to bathing, emphasizing purification and relaxation. The baths become a sanctuary where the rituals of cleansing are intertwined with cultural reverence.

Candlelit Atmosphere:
One of the distinctive features of Hammam Al Ándalus is its candlelit atmosphere. The subdued lighting creates an intimate and serene ambiance, transporting visitors to a time when the soft glow of candles illuminated the bathing chambers.

The flickering light enhances the overall sense of tranquility, allowing patrons to immerse themselves in a meditative experience.

Aromatherapy and Essential Oils:
Hammam Al Ándalus elevates the bathing experience through aromatherapy and the use of essential oils. The air is infused with scents reminiscent of the Mediterranean, enhancing relaxation and promoting a sensory journey. The carefully selected oils contribute to the overall sense of well-being, creating a holistic and aromatic retreat within the historic walls of the baths.

Tea and Relaxation:
After the rejuvenating bath circuit, patrons are invited to indulge in a moment of relaxation. The tea room, adorned with traditional Andalusian decor, becomes a space where visitors can savor herbal teas and reflect on their spa journey. The post-bathing ritual is an essential part of the Hammam Al Ándalus experience, allowing patrons to extend the sense of tranquility beyond the bathing chambers.

Historical and Cultural Context:
Hammam Al Ándalus doesn't just offer a spa experience; it provides a glimpse into Andalusia's historical and cultural context. The baths are situated in proximity to historical landmarks, echoing the region's rich past. This connection to history transforms the spa visit into a cultural pilgrimage, where patrons not only pamper themselves but also immerse in the heritage of Al-Andalus.

Integration with Local Communities:
Each Hammam Al Ándalus location seamlessly integrates with the local communities of Granada, Córdoba, and Málaga. The spa becomes a cultural hub, hosting events, live performances, and workshops that celebrate the diverse traditions of Andalusia. This integration fosters a sense of community and ensures that the baths are not isolated experiences but vibrant contributors to the cultural tapestry of each city.

Holistic Well-Being:
Hammam Al Ándalus, with its emphasis on traditional Arabic baths, architectural allure, and cultural resonance, transcends the typical spa visit. It becomes a holistic well-being experience where patrons engage not only with the waters but also with the centuries-old traditions that have shaped Andalusian culture. As visitors immerse themselves in the soothing embrace of the baths, they embark on a journey that transcends time, offering a taste of Al-Andalusian serenity and cultural richness.

JAPAN.

Takaragawa Onsen - Japan: Mountain Serenity and Open-Air Thermal Bliss

Nestled in the heart of the Japanese mountains, Takaragawa Onsen is a haven for those seeking a unique and rejuvenating experience. Renowned for its outdoor hot spring baths and captivating setting, this *onsen* beckons visitors to immerse themselves in the healing waters while surrounded by the beauty of nature.

Mountainous Retreat:
Takaragawa Onsen is not just a place to soak; it's a mountainous retreat where visitors escape the hustle and bustle of urban life. The *onsen* is situated amidst lush greenery, framed by towering peaks that create a sense of isolation and tranquility. The journey to Takaragawa Onsen becomes a prelude to the serenity that awaits, winding through scenic landscapes and embracing the notion of being one with nature.

Outdoor Hot Spring Baths:
The centerpiece of Takaragawa Onsen's allure is its outdoor hot spring baths, or rotenburo. Scattered along the banks of the Takaragawa River, these baths provide an immersive experience where visitors can submerge themselves in the thermal waters while being enveloped by the crisp mountain air. The open-air setting enhances the connection to nature, making each bath a sensory journey that extends beyond the warmth of the waters.

Picturesque Riverside Setting:
The *onsen's* location along the Takaragawa River adds to its picturesque charm. The soothing sounds of flowing water complement the ambiance, creating a harmonious symphony that enhances the overall experience. Visitors can choose to bathe in pools positioned along the riverbanks, offering panoramic views of the surrounding mountains, making the onsen a visual feast for the senses.

Seasonal Delights:
Takaragawa Onsen transforms with the seasons, providing a different experience throughout the year. In winter, the outdoor baths offer a unique juxtaposition of steaming hot waters against a backdrop of snow-covered landscapes. Spring brings cherry blossoms, and autumn bathers are treated to a kaleidoscope of vibrant colors as the foliage changes. The *onsen* becomes a living canvas that evolves with the natural rhythms of the mountain environment.

Tradition and Simplicity:
The *onsen* experience at Takaragawa is rooted in tradition and simplicity. The focus is on the natural thermal waters and the serene surroundings. Visitors are transported to a time when *onsen* bathing was a meditative practice, a moment to appreciate the healing powers of the Earth and find solace in the mountains. The *onsen's* design and atmosphere pay homage to this simplicity, creating an authentic and unpretentious retreat.

Cultural Connection:
Takaragawa Onsen offers more than just a physical retreat; it provides a cultural connection to Japan's centuries-old *onsen* traditions. The reverence for the natural elements, the emphasis on simplicity, and the integration with the surrounding landscape echo the essence of Japanese *onsen* culture. Visitors become participants in a ritual that transcends the individual bath and becomes a cultural immersion into the art of Japanese relaxation.

Accommodations in Nature:
Beyond the onsen experience, Takaragawa Onsen offers accommodations that seamlessly blend with the natural surroundings. Traditional *ryokan*-style rooms with tatami mat flooring and futon beds provide a serene and comfortable space, further enhancing the overall retreat. The lodgings become an extension of the mountainous landscape, creating a holistic experience that combines comfort with the rustic beauty of the outdoors.

In essence, Takaragawa Onsen is a testament to the transformative power of nature and thermal waters. As visitors soak in the outdoor baths, surrounded by the majesty of the mountains, they embark on a journey that transcends relaxation—it becomes a communion with the elemental forces of Earth and water. Takaragawa Onsen stands as a sanctuary where simplicity, tradition, and nature converge, offering a timeless retreat for those seeking a profound connection with the Japanese mountains and the healing embrace of its hot spring waters.

LONDON.

The Bulgari Spa - London, UK: Opulence and Tranquility in the Heart of the City

Nestled in the vibrant heart of London, The Bulgari Spa emerges as a beacon of luxury, offering a lavish retreat amid the urban bustle. With a plethora of opulent amenities, including a steam room and vitality pool, this spa transcends the conventional, providing a haven of tranquility where the city's rhythm fades away, and indulgence takes center stage.

Urban Oasis:

The Bulgari Spa is more than a mere escape; it's an urban oasis where the tumult of London dissipates, and serenity prevails. Located within the prestigious Bulgari Hotel, the spa seamlessly integrates with the cosmopolitan surroundings while offering an exclusive refuge for those seeking respite from the demands of city life.

Architectural Elegance:

Step into The Bulgari Spa, and you are greeted by architectural elegance that mirrors the sophistication of the Bulgari brand. The design is a harmonious fusion of contemporary chic and classic luxury, creating an ambiance that exudes opulence. Every detail, from the plush furnishings to the carefully curated decor, contributes to an atmosphere of refined indulgence.

Luxurious Spa Facilities:

The Bulgari Spa is a sanctuary where luxury meets wellness. Its facilities are a testament to the commitment to pampering and rejuvenation. The steam room, enveloped in a gentle mist, becomes a retreat for relaxation, detoxification, and skin purification. The vitality pool, with its soothing hydrotherapy jets, invites patrons to immerse themselves in a sensory journey that revitalizes both body and spirit.

Vast Treatment Menu:

Beyond the exceptional facilities, The Bulgari Spa offers a vast menu of treatments designed to cater to the diverse needs of its clientele. From indulgent massages to rejuvenating facials, each treatment is meticulously crafted to enhance well-being and deliver a bespoke spa experience. Highly skilled therapists curate personalized journeys that align with the individual preferences of each guest.

Private Spa Suites:

For those seeking an elevated level of exclusivity, The Bulgari Spa features private spa suites. These intimate retreats provide a secluded space for personalized treatments, ensuring an intimate and tailored experience. The private spa suites embody the pinnacle of luxury, allowing guests to immerse themselves in opulence away from the public spaces.

Cityscape Views:

While enveloped in the luxury of The Bulgari Spa, guests are treated to stunning cityscape views. Floor-to-ceiling windows frame the dynamic city below, creating a captivating backdrop for relaxation. The juxtaposition of the urban panorama against the tranquility of the spa adds a unique dimension to the experience, connecting patrons with the vibrant energy of London.

Holistic Well-Being:
The Bulgari Spa transcends the conventional notion of a spa, embodying a philosophy of holistic well-being. It's not just a place for treatments; it's a retreat for the mind, body, and soul. The meticulous attention to detail, the fusion of opulence and wellness, and the integration of cutting-edge facilities culminate in a spa experience that goes beyond the physical—a journey towards total rejuvenation.

Exclusivity and Accessibility:
While The Bulgari Spa exudes exclusivity, it remains accessible to both guests of the Bulgari Hotel and discerning day visitors. This balance between exclusivity and accessibility ensures that the spa remains a coveted destination for both London residents and international travelers seeking the epitome of luxury in the heart of the city.

In essence, The Bulgari Spa in London transcends the boundaries of traditional spa experiences, redefining opulence and relaxation. As patrons immerse themselves in the steam room, indulge in the vitality pool, and succumb to bespoke treatments, they embark on a journey where luxury intertwines with tranquility, creating an unparalleled haven in the heart of one of the world's most dynamic cities.

AUSTRALIA.

The Peninsula Hot Springs - Australia: Geothermal Bliss in Natural Splendor

Nestled in the picturesque landscapes of Victoria, Australia, The Peninsula Hot Springs beckon visitors to embark on a journey of relaxation and rejuvenation amidst geothermal wonders. Renowned for its geothermal pools and spa experiences, this haven of tranquility seamlessly blends the therapeutic benefits of thermal waters with the breathtaking beauty of the natural surroundings.

Natural Setting and Geothermal Pools:
The Peninsula Hot Springs present a rare fusion of natural beauty and geothermal marvels. Surrounded by lush greenery and overlooking the scenic landscape, the geothermal pools become a focal point for visitors seeking solace and serenity. These pools, heated by the Earth's natural heat, offer a unique bathing experience that goes beyond relaxation—it becomes a communion with the Earth's elemental forces.

Variety of Bathing Experiences:
The Peninsula Hot Springs cater to a diverse range of preferences with a variety

of bathing experiences. From communal thermal pools where socializing becomes a part of the relaxation to private baths that offer secluded indulgence, visitors can tailor their experience to suit their desires. Each pool, with its unique temperature and ambiance, provides a distinct sensory journey.

Hilltop Pool with Panoramic Views:
One of the highlights of The Peninsula Hot Springs is the Hilltop Pool, perched strategically to offer panoramic views of the surrounding landscape. As patrons soak in the warm waters, they are treated to a visual feast of rolling hills, tranquil lakes, and native flora. The Hilltop Pool becomes a vantage point where the therapeutic benefits of geothermal bathing harmonize with the scenic beauty of the Australian countryside.

Cave Pool for Subterranean Serenity:
Adding to the diversity of experiences, the Cave Pool at The Peninsula Hot Springs offers a subterranean retreat. Set within a cave-like enclave, this pool provides a sense of seclusion and mystery. The ambient lighting and natural rock formations create an intimate atmosphere, transporting bathers to an otherworldly sanctuary beneath the Earth's surface.

Turkish Steam Bath and Saunas:
Beyond the geothermal pools, The Peninsula Hot Springs offer Turkish steam baths and a range of saunas. These spaces become sanctuaries of heat-induced relaxation, promoting detoxification and enhancing overall well-being. The combination of geothermal waters and heat therapies creates a holistic approach to rejuvenation, catering to both the physical and mental aspects of wellness.

Natural Thermal Mud:
The spa experiences at The Peninsula Hot Springs extend beyond water therapies. The presence of natural thermal mud encourages visitors to indulge in a unique form of skincare. The mineral-rich mud, sourced from the geothermal waters, is believed to have nourishing and revitalizing properties. Guests can engage in a self-applied mud ritual, enhancing their spa journey with the Earth's natural gifts.

Connection to Aboriginal Culture:
The Peninsula Hot Springs honor and celebrate the rich Aboriginal culture of the region. The spa experiences are influenced by traditional Aboriginal bathing practices, creating a respectful connection to the land's indigenous heritage. Visitors not only enjoy the therapeutic benefits of the geothermal waters but also partake in a cultural immersion that adds depth to their spa experience.

Wellness Beyond Soaking:
The Peninsula Hot Springs embrace a holistic approach to wellness, extending beyond the act of soaking in thermal waters. The spa offers a range of wellness activities, including yoga classes and meditation sessions. These activities become integral components of the overall experience, allowing patrons to nurture their minds and bodies in harmony with the natural surroundings.

Sustainability and Environmental Stewardship:
In addition to providing a haven for relaxation, The Peninsula Hot Springs are committed to sustainability and environmental stewardship. The spa is designed to minimize its ecological footprint, incorporating eco-friendly practices and initiatives. This commitment to environmental responsibility enhances the overall experience, allowing visitors to connect with nature while knowing that their wellness journey aligns with principles of conservation.

The Peninsula Hot Springs in Australia transcend the traditional spa experience. As visitors immerse themselves in the geothermal pools, caves, and saunas, they embark on a journey that harmonizes the healing powers of thermal waters with the untouched beauty of the Australian landscape. The Peninsula Hot Springs become a sanctuary where relaxation, cultural respect, and environmental mindfulness converge, offering a holistic retreat for those seeking the transformative embrace of nature's geothermal wonders.

FINAL THOUGHTS

In the dimming glow of this exploration into the history and health benefits of saunas and steam, one is left to ponder the profound tapestry woven by time, tradition, and well-being. This narrative, a voyage across the ages, has laid bare the roots of these ancient practices, showcasing their enduring relevance in the human experience.

As we traverse the pages, we find ourselves immersed in the cultural narratives of diverse civilizations, each contributing threads to the evolution of sauna and steam bathing. From the rustic saunas of Finnish landscapes to the ornate hammams of the Middle East, the cultural diversity encapsulated within these sanctuaries resonates with the universal human pursuit of repose, purification, and shared connection.

The interplay of history and health unfolds like a well-choreographed dance, revealing the mysteries shrouded within the swirling steam and embracing warmth. The scientific revelations about the therapeutic virtues of sauna and steam baths bridge the chasm between tradition and contemporary wellness, offering a glimpse into the physiological wonders these practices bestow on the body and soul.

This narrative isn't merely an account of facts; it's an invitation to partake in the sauna and steam rituals firsthand. The vivid descriptions beckon the reader into the heart of steamy chambers, where the heat enfolds the body, and tranquility becomes a companion. Whether exploring the humble wood-fired saunas of secluded retreats or luxuriating in the opulent steam rooms of urban spas, the narrative is a guide, urging readers to embark on their wellness journey.

As the curtain falls on these pages, the narrative transcends its role as a historical and scientific exploration, morphing into a call for the continued reverence and preservation of these timeless traditions. The cultural legacy and the role of saunas and steam in fostering communal bonds come to the forefront. Readers are left with a deep appreciation for the ancient wisdom passed down through generations and a heightened awareness of the pivotal role saunas and steam play in modern-day wellness practices.

In essence, as we bid adieu to this narrative, we carry not just knowledge but a profound appreciation for the rituals that have withstood the test of time. The history and health benefits of sauna and steam have been laid bare, and the journey within these pages echoes the timeless call to step into the comforting arms of steam, to savor the warmth that transcends centuries, and to immerse ourselves in the profound well-being that beckons within the steam-filled chambers of tradition and science.

Afterword:

As you close the pages of "Steam & Sauna: A Concise Guidebook," I invite you to embark on a personal journey that extends beyond the words on these pages. Saunas and steam have an incredible way of weaving themselves into the fabric of our lives, creating experiences that transcend the ordinary.

Consider this not just a book but a key to unlock a world of warmth, wellness, and exploration. Whether you're a seasoned sauna enthusiast or a newcomer, your journey with saunas and steam is a lifetime adventure. It's about more than just the heat; it's about the places you'll go, the people you'll meet, and the stories you'll share.

As you venture into saunas and steam rooms, whether in your travels or within the comfort of your home, keep a journal or jot down notes. Chronicle your experiences, the places you visit, the friendships forged in the soothing embrace of steam, and the moments of profound relaxation and revelation.

Your journey with saunas and steam is unique and personal. It's about creating a tapestry of memories that will stay with you for a lifetime. Let this book be the starting point, the inspiration for a lifetime of experiences with the power of heat.

Before you close this chapter, I'd like to share a little more about SaunaFin, the industry leader that ignited this journey from a casual interest to a consuming and life-affirming passion. For well over six decades, SaunaFin has been a venerable guide in the realm of custom steam and sauna solutions. From its inception in 1962 as Finlanda Sauna, the commitment has been unwavering – to refine the craftsmanship that goes into constructing saunas, each a testament to a storied heritage.

SaunaFin seamlessly intertwines ancient traditions with cutting-edge technology, creating a harmonious synthesis that transcends time. The metamorphosis to SaunaFin in 1996 symbolized a dedication to evolution and innovation, distinguishing itself in craftsmanship and custom solutions.

Beyond being manufacturers, SaunaFin sees themselves as custodians of well-being, recognizing that the allure of a sauna extends beyond its physical confines. They don't just construct saunas; they weave spaces echoing the harmony of tradition and innovation.

As SaunaFin is proud to support this exploration of steam and sauna traditions, their commitment to preserving ancient traditions and illuminating the evolution of steam and sauna experiences is evident. Through their dedication and the highest quality materials, they aim to foster a deeper understanding of the therapeutic and cultural aspects of steam and sauna rituals.

Now, as you continue your journey, remember that every steam session and sauna visit is a new chapter waiting to be written. So, keep notes, collect memories, and savor the warmth of each moment. Your journey with saunas and steam is a lifelong story, and the pages are yours to fill.

Warm regards,

Alberto Rossi
11/2023